authentic aromatherapy

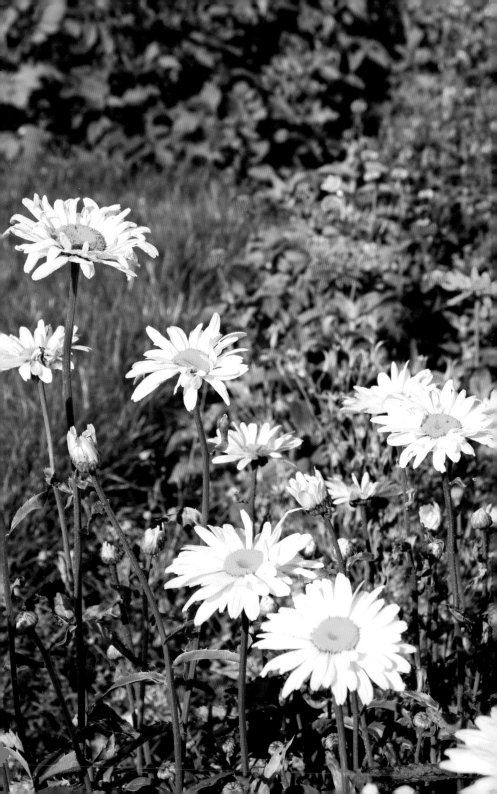

authentic aromatherapy

Essential Oils and Blends for Health, Beauty, and Home

Sharon Falsetto

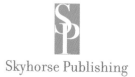

Skyhorse Publishing

Skyhorse Publishing books may be purchased in bulk at special discounts for sales promotion, corporate gifts, fund-raising, or educational purposes. Special editions can also be created to specifications. For details, contact the Special Sales Department, Skyhorse Publishing, 307 West 36th Street, 11th Floor, New York, NY 10018 or info@skyhorsepublishing.com.

Skyhorse® and Skyhorse Publishing® are registered trademarks of Skyhorse Publishing, Inc.®, a Delaware corporation.

www.skyhorsepublishing.com

10 9 8 7 6 5 4 3 2 1

Library of Congress Cataloging-in-Publication Data is available on file.

ISBN: 978-1-62636-415-8

Printed in China

For my grandmother, Eva

contents

Part Three: Essential Oils Reference Guide – 149

Disclaimer

The information provided in this book is intended for your personal learning experience and does not endorse or advocate the use of a particular product or service mentioned here within. The author does not guarantee the outcome of the use of essential oils, as outlined in this book, and is not licensed to diagnose or claim to cure any health concerns, where mentioned. Although every effort has been made to ensure that the information supplied is correct, to the best of the author's knowledge, the author does not take responsibility for how you use the information in this book.

This book is not intended to replace professional training but is intended to be a general guide to those seeking information about the subject matter. The information given in this book relates to the external use of essential oils and does not extensively cover either the internal use of essential oils, or the use of herbs and other plants in herbal medicine, where outcomes might be different.

In addition, none of the statements within this book have been endorsed by the U.S. Food and Drug Administration or any government agency worldwide. The author and publisher do not take any responsibility or hold any liability for the use, or misuse, of the information provided, which might result in injury or damage to people or property. This book is not a substitute for medical advice from your health practitioner, and you are advised to seek medical assistance, or the advice of a certified and experienced professional aromatherapist, where appropriate, before using the information supplied in this book.

About the Book

Authentic Aromatherapy is written as a complete handbook for the beginner to aromatherapy, in an attempt to demystify the business of aromatherapy and essential oils, and to introduce you to the many different ways in which you can use essential oils in your home. It is a simple introduction for either the professional or lay person new to aromatherapy.

Authentic Aromatherapy is split into three main sections. *Part One: The Basics of Essential Oils* covers the history of using scents and healing plants, the difference between essential oils, fragrance oils, and other plant extracts, the quality of essential oils, and how essential oils are extracted. There is also information on the basic chemistry of essential oils.

Part Two: Using Essential Oils covers how essential oils work and the many different ways in which you can use essential oils safely for yourself and in your home. *Part Three: Essential Oils Reference Guide* introduces you to profiles of forty essential oils suitable for using in the ways discussed in *Part Two*.

Authentic Aromatherapy is designed to be read as a whole, but the three individual sections make it easy for you to refer back to a particular essential oil, or section, time and time again, as needed.

It is my hope that *Authentic Aromatherapy* will prove to be a comprehensive introduction to essential oils and be the start of your journey into the world of aromatherapy! There is so much more information that I could have included in this book, but I think you will find that the book is an adequate reference to begin your journey. If it helps you to demystify one piece of information, or introduces you to one new way of using essential oils, it has been worth my journey in writing it.

Introduction

Aromatherapy is a practice that is often thought of as nothing more than a way of producing pleasing aromas. However, it is so much more than this! Plant extracts and scent have a long history of use—both as a cosmetic and a medicinal tool—but it is only in modern day history that interest in aromatherapy has begun to grow again.

Aromatherapy as a therapy is often misunderstood, given that the broad term *aromatherapy* is sometimes misused both in the aromatherapy industry and in general. *Aromatherapy* is a word that is used to describe anything from a true essential oil candle to a commercial air freshener. However, these two products couldn't be more different, in source, chemical makeup, and benefits.

I did not truly understand these differences myself until I embarked on my professional studies in aromatherapy several years ago. Since then, I have relocated from one country (the United Kingdom) to another (the United States) and learned how people view the business of aromatherapy, through different eyes in different places.

Along the way, I have had the good fortune to be tutored by several great teachers—in one way or another—and have had the opportunity to study the source of essential oils and the plants themselves, up close and personal in France. However, it is perhaps the customers and students whom I encounter in my day-to-day business who have led me to understand and appreciate the many different ways in which you can use essential oils, through their various requests and questions.

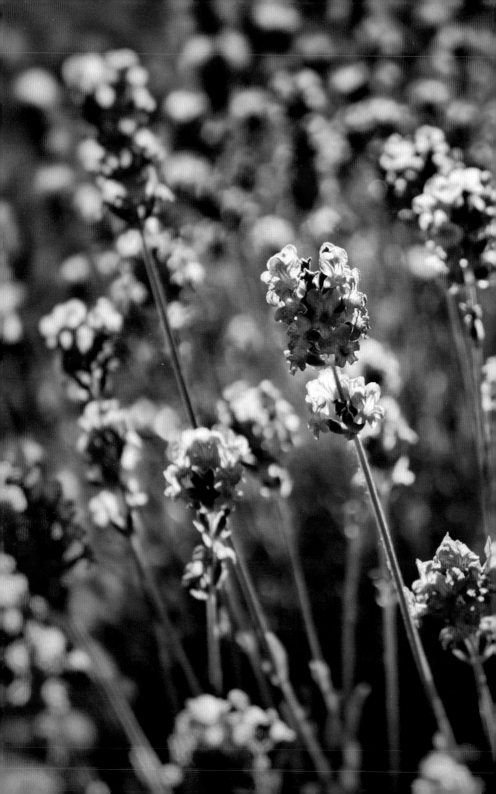

Part One

The Basics of Essential Oils

I

Brief History of Scents and Use of Healing Plants

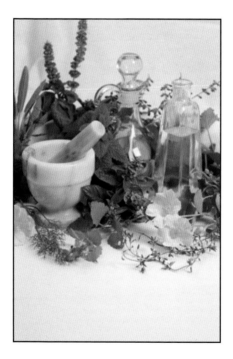

Ancient History

Many trace the history of aromatherapy back to ancient civilizations in India, China, and Egypt. Although an essential oil, as we know it today, was not used *per se* by such civilizations, it is true

that such civilizations extensively used plants to create medicinal remedies and perfumed cosmetics. It is the historic use of
these plants and scents that is covered in this chapter.

Ancient India
Due to the absence of accurate record keeping, India holds
perhaps one of the oldest records for medicinal use of aromatic
plants. Although it is likely that aromatic plants were in use
before such time, the Indian book of *Vedas* dates back to approximately 2000 BC. This ancient book lists over seven hundred
plants, including sandalwood, myrrh, and cinnamon.

Ancient China
The ancient Chinese also used plants medicinally. One of the
oldest Chinese records on medicine, *The Yellow Emperor's Book of
Internal Medicine*, dates back to approximately 2000 BC. Ginger is
mentioned as part of a therapeutic remedy in this book.

Ancient Egypt
People of ancient Egypt were among one of the first civilizations to realize the many uses of healing plants. In addition,
the ancient Egyptians kept various records of their findings and
plant use, making such information accessible to people today.
They not only used the plant itself for various ailments and religious practices, but the oil extracted from such a plant was used
to heal, perfume, and beautify, too. Ancient Egyptians did not
use the same extraction methods as those used today to extract an
oil from a plant, but they were not too dissimilar. Over time, the
process evolved into the current distillation method to produce
essential oils.

The Egyptians had access to and the means for growing many of the healing aromatic plants that they used in everyday life. The fertile plains of the river Nile provided a rich growing area for several aromatic plants, including those that the Egyptians imported from exotic lands such as Persia and Syria. Persia was home to the biblical Hanging Gardens of Babylon, a lush paradise of fragrant trees, flowers, and herbs. Fragrant trees and plants, such as sandalwood, myrrh, frankincense, and labdanum populated the valley around the river Nile that soon became known as the "cradle of medicine." Both the ancient Greeks and Romans traveled to Egypt to learn about the Egyptians' aromatic treasure chest.

Healing plants and scents played a dominant role in an ancient Egyptian's life. Scents were used for sacred and religious celebrations, in addition to cosmetic and therapeutic uses. Scents were extracted from plants like myrrh, juniper, and saffron and offered in honor of gods in the ancient temples. In death, bodies were mummified with plant scents to help ensure an everlasting life.

Hieroglyphics in temples such as those at Edfu present evidence of the use of aromatic plants in ancient Egypt. Edfu also contains the description of one of the most famous Egyptian perfumes, *Kyphi*. The exact ingredients of *Kyphi* are open to interpretation, depending upon which text you read, but *Kyphi* was reputed to ease anxiety and promote sleep, among other ailments. Essences such as *Kyphi* were used both as a perfume and a medicine, in addition to embalming bodies after death.

The ancient King Tutankhamen's tomb presents evidence of both the use and the antiseptic qualities of Egyptian aromatic resins and oils. When the tomb was opened 3,000 years after King

Tutankhamen's death, the aroma of frankincense and myrrh was still evident. Further evidence of ancient Egyptian plant use is also found in the *Ebers Papyrus*. *The Ebers Papyrus* is one of the earliest Egyptian records of medicinal plant use and gives an insight into the ancient Egyptian world of aromatic plants. Although the *Ebers Papyrus* dates back to 1550 BC, it wasn't discovered until 1873 by the Egyptologist Ebers. It contains about one hundred medicinal prescriptions, including familiar aromatic plant names that we know and use today.

Ancient Greece

Ancient Greeks who visited the area known as the "cradle of medicine" were greatly impressed with what they saw and learned from the Egyptians, and took this knowledge back home with them. Among those Greek visitors was a physician by the name of Hippocrates (460 BC–370 BC). Hippocrates helped to establish a medical school on the Greek island of Kos as a result of his visits to Egypt and the knowledge that he learned there. Hippocrates earned the name "Father of Medicine" because of his contribution to the field of medicine.

Legend tells that Hippocrates taught his students about medicinal plants and herbs beneath the shade of a large plane tree; a plane tree still stands in this spot today (although it is not the original tree). This area, which I visited many years ago, is popular with visitors today, due in part to this legend. Hippocrates' teachings are recorded in a collection of approximately seventy medicinal works, collectively referred to as *Corpus Hippocraticum*, although it is commonly believed that Hippocrates himself was not responsible for the full content of this work; it is believed that the collection contained the work of his students and followers, too.

Hippocrates was not the only famous Greek of his time: a Greek named Megallus was responsible for formulating a perfume from aromatic substances that became known by the name *Megaleion*. *Megaleion* was as popular in its time as some of the more famous perfumes today. Reputedly it had healing properties that reduced inflammation and helped heal wounds. In addition, a Greek physician by the name of Peodanius Dioscorides (40 AD–90 AD) wrote a book entitled *De Materia Medica*, which became a precursor to modern day pharmacopoeias.

Like the Egyptians, the Greeks used scent as part of their everyday life for beauty and hygienic purposes and for the celebration of birth, marriage, and death. They used oils with a base of iris, rose, marjoram, and lily. Other precious essences included myrrh, incense, saffron, and cinnamon. Scented oils were used in Greek society as testimony to the height of good hospitality—scenting the hair with oil and washing the feet with oil were both common practices.

Even Greek soldiers saw the benefit of perfumes, oils, and creams made from plants. They used them to protect themselves from the intense sun and to help with hygiene issues. Aromatic oils were also used to treat battle wounds.

The ancient Greeks classified and recorded the botanical and aromatic knowledge that they had learned from the ancient Egyptians, which in turn influenced the Romans' growing appreciation of aromatic plants.

Ancient Rome and Pompeii Use

The ancient Romans attached great importance to the use of plants and scents. Due to the vastness of the Roman empire, knowledge about the use of healing plants spread far and wide.

Herbs such as rosemary, thyme, and fennel made their way across borders with the Roman armies and were introduced to countries like Great Britain where these plants still thrive today in many gardens.

The Romans were famous for using aromatic plants and perfumes to excess, utilizing them in the hosting of extravagant banquets and in the Roman baths. Eventually, by 1 BC, the Romans attributed a specific scent or plant to every God, such as amber to Venus and cinnamon to Mercury.

Situated to the south of Rome was the city of Pompeii, which was also no stranger to the use of aromatic plants. Pompeii disappeared under a huge pile of lava and ash during the eruption of nearby volcano, Mount Vesuvius, in 79 AD. We know much about how the people of ancient Pompeii used plants and perfumes due to the remarkable preservation of the city. Modern day archaeologists unearthed much evidence in excavations of the ancient city that showed the extent to which the Pompeians used aromatic plants. Because ancient Pompeii was situated beneath the fertile slopes of Mount Vesuvius, it was extremely favorable for growing many plants, including rose, myrtle, and laurel.

Ancient frescoes found in the House of Vettii depict the collections of plants and flowers and the process of perfume making. Pompeian ladies used aromatic plants for perfumes and cosmetic lotions that also had medicinal uses. Some of those recipes are recorded in various books and records of that time (such as Pliny's in *Naturalis Historia* and Discorides' in *De Materia Medica*). For those of us who don't have access to these great works, books such as *Profumi, Ungenti e Acconciature in Pompei Antica* (*Perfumes, Ungents and Hairstyles in Pompeii*) by Carlo Giordano and Angelandrea Casale summarize ancient perfume recipes such as these (note that the actual recipes may have included other plant ingredients, too):

- *Mirtum-Laurum*—laurel, myrtle, myrrh, and lily
- *Rhodimum*— rose, fennel, and myrrh
- *Susinum*—honey, myrrh, saffron, lily, and cinnamon

If you visit the archaeological site of ancient Pompeii today, as I did several years ago, you can see some of this evidence first hand. It is a fascinating insight into a world that was essentially lost for centuries.

Early Distillation

One of the greatest contributors to the world of modern day essential oil distillation was a physician from Persia by the name of Avicenna (980 AD–1037 AD), also known by the name Ib'n Sina. Avicenna drew much of his knowledge of medicine from Greek, Chinese, and Ayurvedic medicine, including that of Hippocrates. Avicenna wrote the medicinal text, *Canon of Medicine*, which was studied by many Medieval medicine students. However, although Avicenna's knowledge of medicine, and particularly that of medicinal plants, was remarkable, it was his invention of the refrigerated coil in the distillation of plants for which he is historically remembered.

Although it is known that ancient civilizations, such as the Egyptians, were using some form of distillation before Avicenna's invention, it was the addition of a refrigerated coil that improved the entire process. Avicenna reputedly distilled rose as one of the first plants in the new distillation process. Interestingly, before the introduction of the refrigerated coil, essential oils were more often than not seen as a by-product of the whole process, with favor given to the aromatic waters produced (or hydrosols as we know them today).

Medieval Herbals and Practices

Aromatic plants found their way into Medieval Europe with the Crusades (a series of Holy Wars between the Saracens and the Europeans (1095–1291), and through the spice routes, as the gap between East and West was bridged. Although the ancient Greeks and Romans originally carried the knowledge of aromatic plant medicine back from Egypt, much of it was lost during a period of time dubbed as the Dark Ages. However, some of this knowledge was preserved on isolated islands in the Mediterranean, where the Crusaders rediscovered it on their way home.

Medieval monasteries were popular places for aromatic herb gardens, and plants such as thyme, lavender, and rosemary flourished. Cloister gardens established within the sacred walls of the monastery were split into physics gardens, for medicinal purposes, and kitchen gardens, for culinary purposes.

During the fourteenth century, the Black Death (or Bubonic Plague) raged throughout Europe. Many aromatic spices and herbs were used in the fight of this deadly disease: frankincense was one of several plants burned in the streets or worn around the neck to protect people from the Black Death.

During medieval times, understanding and knowledge of medicinal plants increased through the research of physician and botanist Paracelsus (1493–1541), and Medieval herbals written by English herbalist John Gerard (1545–1612) and physician Nicholas Culpeper (1616–1654). Voyages into the new world helped to increase the knowledge of many medicinal plants.

The Passion for French Scents

France had several popular figures who helped to promote the use of scents and healing plants. A couple of French queens appear to have had a connection with scent in one way or another. Catherine de Medici (1519–1589) was the queen consort of France from 1547 to 1559, and wife of King Henry II of France. Catherine de Medici is said to have instigated the growing of the many fragrant flowers suitable to the Mediterranean climate of Grasse (in southern France), based on the knowledge that she brought with her from her native Italy. The perfumery industry that evolved into the one in Grasse today is a result of these early beginnings.

Queen Marie Antoinette of France (1755–1793) also had an interest in scent, aside from her infamous passion for fashion. She had her own personal perfumer, Jean-Louis Fargeon (1748–1806), who created many perfumes and scents exclusively for the French queen. Jean-Louis Fargeon created many perfumes, including one known as the *Parfum de Trianon*. Some of the ingredients were violet, rose, jonquil, tuberose, amber, and opopanax.

Fargeon also made many medicinal and aromatic remedies for Marie Antoinette's bath and boudoir and for her pregnancies. Ultimately, Marie Antoinette's love of her favorite perfumes and aromatic remedies may have cost her her life. According to Elisabeth de Feydeau in *A Scented Palace*, Marie Antoinette's insistence on waiting for her favorite perfumes to be made for her, prior to her attempt to flee France during the French Revolution (1789–1799), delayed her departure. She was executed on October 16, 1793.

Modern-Day Aromatherapy

The use of aromatic plants declined in countries such as Great Britain as the industrial revolution (1760–1840/1850) took hold. People deserted their country homes in favor of work in the cities, where gardens (and space for growing plants) were sparse. The development of synthetic drugs also contributed to people's abandonment of medicinal plants. The use of true medicinal plants and the scents extracted from them was, for the most part, forgotten.

However, during the late nineteenth and early part of the twentieth century, the revival in medicinal plant use and the advancement to the use of essential oils began, through the hard work, research, and advocacy of pioneers such as René-Maurice Gattefossé (1881–1950), Marguerite Maury (1895–1968), Jean Valnet (1920–1995), Robert Tisserand, and Shirley Price.

Perhaps the most famous aromatherapy tales of these modern day pioneers belong to Gattefossé. Gattefossé is a name that is familiar to all aromatherapy students today, although the exact sequence of events that is often told regarding Gattefossé's infamous "discovery" of the benefits of lavender essential oil is sometimes misconfabulated. He was a French chemist and scientist whose family was heavily involved in the aromatic plant and perfume industry, including those essences known as essential oils. Gattefossé allegedly used essential oils for the treatment of wounds during his military service in World War I (1914–1918). He is accredited for coming up with the modern day term and use of the word *aromathérapie* through his work in the family perfumery business. It was an attempt to separate the medicinal properties of essential oils from the common use of oils in perfumery.

The popular story of Gattefossé's discovery of the healing benefits of lavender essential oil goes as follows: Gattefossé plunged his hand into a vat of lavender after an experiment did not go according to plan. His hand did not bear the burn scarring that it would have done if left untreated.

Each civilization over time attached a different significance to aromatic plants and scents, despite their many uses. In ancient Egypt, scent was very much revered through religious practices. The Romans used scent often as a status symbol. French queens and nobility had access to some of the finest resources for making aromatic perfumes and potions. In Great Britain, it used to be common to find aromatic plants in nearly every country cottage garden, making such "medicine" available to all.

Today, aromatherapy is used in clinical and holistic settings to help with various health problems, as an integrative therapy with practices such as massage, reflexology, and reiki, and it is a term that is applied to many natural body care products. The true practice of aromatherapy uses essential oils, not fragrance oils: The ways in which to use these essential oils are discussed in *Part Two*.

2

Essential Oils vs. Fragrance Oils

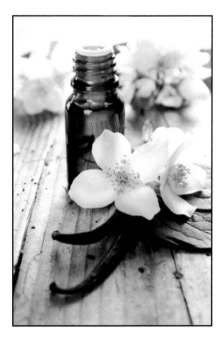

The commercial use of the word *aromatherapy* has led to several misunderstandings as to the use of essential oils in aromatherapy practice. Although the word *aromatherapy* is used to describe all types of fragrant products, essential oils are the only true products that are extracted from plants (aside from such products as absolutes and resins, as discussed in chapter 4).

Although essential oils and fragrance oils can sometimes be used for the same purpose, they are chemically different, priced differently, and possess different properties; fragrance oils do not possess therapeutic properties. The popular use of fragrance oils in the growing bath and body industry has contributed further to the confusion between the oils. This chapter attempts to explain the differences between the two types of oils.

Defining an Essential Oil

An essential oil is a substance that is extracted from a plant in a number of ways (as discussed in chapter 5). Not all plants contain an essential oil, an important distinction to remember when questioning if it is possible to extract an essential oil from, for example, a strawberry (it is not).

Essential oils are obtained from the roots, flowers, leaves, seeds, and bark of a plant. A pure essential oil is obtained from a single plant species, although there might be various chemo-types of one particular essential oil or a blending of essential oils in a distilled mix. It is the "aroma" of the plant (stored in the tiny glands, sacs, and hairs) that is captured in an essential oil and used therapeutically in aromatherapy.

Plants that do hold essential oils contain various therapeutic properties that are reputed to help with a number of health ailments. Such essential oils are used in clinical aromatherapy practice to help with difficulties and self body care including physical prob-lems (muscle pain, arthritis, nausea), emotional problems (stress, depression, anxiety), menstrual problems (PMS and menopausal difficulties), and skin care. They also have a wide variety of other uses, as discussed in *Part Two*.

Defining a Fragrance Oil

A fragrance oil is a man-made, synthetic product derived from a chemical combination of substances and put together in a scientific laboratory. It is blended in such a way that it resembles the aroma of a specific plant or product. Some fragrance oils might combine essential oils, too, in their makeup. Fragrance oils do not possess any therapeutic properties; in fact, many people are often allergic to chemical components that go into producing a fragrance oil or perfume.

The majority of modern-day commercial perfumes are synthetically made (although some may also contain a small amount of true essential oils); in the past, perfumes were made with natural plant oils in addition to other animal and plant derivatives.

Essential oils are usually more subtle in aroma, which is one indication as to whether you are dealing with an essential oil or a fragrance oil. It is possible to create almost any aroma in a fragrance oil, unlike an essential oil, which can only be extracted from a plant that actually contains an essential oil.

Chemical Composition of an Essential Oil

An essential oil is complex in chemical composition. For example, rose otto (*Rosa damascena*) essential oil has over three hundred individual chemical components, making it extremely difficult to synthetically duplicate each component in the exact proportions of the essential oil. In fact, scientists are still trying to identify and assess some of the more complex chemical components in essential oils.

Essential oils are volatile substances. The chemical components of essential oils vary in the same species of plant due to season, climate, and growing conditions. This means that the aroma and chemical components of an essential oil can vary slightly between each batch produced. The quality of an essential oil is tested through various means, but these tests can only distinguish a "standard" reading expected of an essential oil drawn from that plant species because of the factors described.

Examples of true essential oils that have been extracted from plants are given in *Part Three*.

Chemical Composition of a Fragrance Oil

A fragrance oil is not a volatile substance because it is synthetically made. Therefore, a fragrance oil will last longer, in fragrance and shelf life, than an essential oil. The shelf life of an essential oil varies between one year for a citrus essential oil, such as grapefruit (*Citrus x paradisi*), to several years for an essential oil such as patchouli (*Pogostemon cablin*).

You will also find a wide range of fragrance oils available. In addition to synthetic duplication of true essential oil aromas, it is also possible to find fragrance oils ranging from plant aromas, such as strawberry, apple, melon, and pineapple (which some mistake for essential oils), to food aromas, such as bacon, blueberry, and hot fudge. Basically, you can almost have any type of aroma you desire in a fragrance oil.

Differences in the Pricing of Essential Oils and Fragrance Oils

Essential oils vary considerably in price depending upon the type of essential oil, season, and availability. However, some essential oils, such as rose otto, are always expensively priced because of the complex extraction process involved. As a guideline, if you find rose essential oil at a cheap price you can probably assume that it is either adulterated or is, in fact, a fragrance oil. Citrus essential oils are usually the lowest priced essential oils because they are relatively easy (and abundant) to extract.

Fragrance oils are much cheaper in price than essential oils because it is a lot easier to produce the same aroma *en masse*. Take, for example, aromatherapy candles: compare a factory-produced candle with a synthetic aroma to a soy-based candle infused with a true essential oil, and you will find that the factory-produced candle is a lot cheaper than the soy-based candle. The factory-produced candle usually contains harmful and cheap ingredients, whereas the essential oil candle contains natural ingredients. Sometimes, you do get exactly what you pay for!

Essential Oil or Fragrance Oil?

Essential oils are used both in the therapeutic practice of aromatherapy and in true aromatherapy skin-care products and candles, as a flavoring in food and alcohol, in natural perfumery, and in soaps and detergents. Fragrance oils are used in many body products, perfumes, and soap but have no therapeutic value in the practice of true aromatherapy.

3

Organic vs. Non-Organic Essential Oils

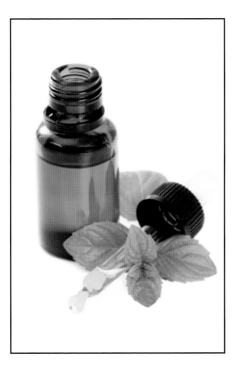

"Essential oils" is a broad term and encompasses organic, non-organic, and wild crafted oils. Wild crafted essential oils are usually handcrafted these days, so you will find that there are two main types of essential oils on the general retail market: organic and non-organic.

Essential oils have to meet certain criteria in order to be legally classified as one type of essential oil or another. Different countries have different types of legislation to comply with; for example, in the United States, the US Department of Agriculture (USDA) governs the laws and regulations regarding organic labeling for products.

Wild Crafted Essential Oils

You probably won't find many true wild crafted essential oils on the market (although there are a few available from select suppliers of essential oils). Wild crafted essential oils are also sometimes extracted at home using a home still. In simple terms, a wild crafted essential oil is obtained from a wild crafted plant. A wild crafted plant is a plant that is found growing naturally in the wild or cultivated—provided that it meets certain criteria. Country regulations vary, but, as a guideline, a wild crafted essential oil has usually been extracted from a plant in its most natural state and/or with minimum farming.

Organic Essential Oils

Today, many products are labeled as "organic." However, this is a broad term that can be interpreted to have various meanings, depending upon the product being discussed. An essential oil that is labeled as organic has to be extracted from a plant that has been grown and farmed organically, following the certification guidelines of the organization from which organic certification is sought.

Organic growing and farming methods restrict the use of artificial chemical fertilizers and pesticides. Plants are also not allowed to be genetically modified. In addition, a farmer has to be certified as an organic farmer to be able to produce plants that will distill organic essential oils. Consequently, organic essential oils are priced higher than non-organic ones due to the higher production and certification costs involved.

USDA Certified Organic

In the United States, farmers and producers of certified organic products have to comply with the USDA National Organic Program (NOP). U.S. organic farming methods exclude the use of synthetic chemicals and hormones in crop production and rely on practices such as biological pest management.

In order to legally use and trade on the USDA certified organic label, a farmer or producer must first comply with USDA organic regulations as specified in the U.S. Code of Federal Regulations (CFR) at 7 (Agriculture) CFR Section 205 of the National Organic Program. A farmer or producer can apply to become "certified organic" if they comply with the regulations as specified, and submit a lengthy application (and a sum of money) to a USDA-accredited certifying agent. USDA-certified organic farmers and producers operate both in the United States and around the world.

Non-Organic Essential Oils

Although a non-organic essential oil is still regarded as a pure essential oil, plants that are grown and farmed non-organically to produce essential oils have usually been treated with pesticides and chemical fertilizers. However, some may argue that only a minuscule amount of chemicals and pesticides are transferred from plant to bottle in the distilling of an essential oil, a subject often open to debate, as it is very difficult to "prove" or "disprove" this point. It is perhaps for this reason that is has become necessary in today's world to "certify" a product as organic, in order to reassure the consumer that certain guidelines have, indeed, been followed.

Organic or Non-Organic?

Both organic and non-organic essential oils have the same therapeutic properties for true aromatherapy practice because they are both extracted from plants (unlike fragrance oils). The chemical composition analysis of an essential oil, established through a test such as GC-MS analysis, will not usually show a difference in the chemical constituents of a particular essential oil, whether it is has been extracted from a plant that is grown organically or non-organically. However, the question is, to what extent has the final essential oil possibly been affected by the different farming and production methods involved in its extraction from the plant? And has this residue left a trace component in the final essential oil (a factor that is not determined via GC-MS analysis)?

Organic essential oils are usually higher priced than non-organic essential oils because of the attention to detail in the farming and extraction of the plant and the costs involved in the certification process. You might ask, is a higher priced organic essential oil worth more, in therapeutic value, than a non-organic essential oil?

Certified organic usually means quality and peace of mind that the essential oil has met stringent criteria for certification. However, it is also equally possible that the farming and extraction methods of a non-organic producer might follow very closely the guidelines for organic essential oil labeling, even though they don't have the official seal of approval. In order to make an informed decision when choosing an organic or non-organic essential oil, get to know, and trust, your essential oil supplier.

4

Hydrosols, Resins, Absolutes, and Carrier Oils

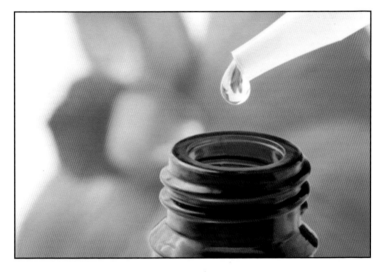

Chapter 2 discussed the differences between essential oils and fragrance oils. To recap, essential oils are natural, whereas fragrance oils are not. However, essential oils are not the only substances that are extracted from plants for use in true aromatherapy practice. Other natural and semi-natural substances are often used for aromatherapy (and perfumery) purposes—these substances include absolutes, resins, hydrosols, and carrier oils.

Some plants produce a variety of different substances for extraction; for example, it is possible for a plant to produce not only an essential oil, but also a hydrosol, absolute, and/or resin. In addition, a plant might produce both a carrier oil and an essential oil, although the essential oil might not always be suitable for therapeutic practice. The almond (*Prunis dulcis*) tree produces both a carrier oil and an essential oil. However, the essential oil is considered too toxic for aromatherapy use. Not all plants are capable of producing all of these substances for extraction purposes, so it is beneficial to understand what each type of extracted substance is and the process for doing so.

Hydrosols: A By-product of Distillation

A hydrosol is an aromatherapy product that has grown in popularity in recent years in the United States, but it is not a new phenomenon. Interestingly, in the early days of plant distillation, it was the hydrosol that was valued more than the essential oil; an essential oil was considered to be the by-product of distillation, not the hydrosol.

In modern times, roles were reversed, and hydrosols became known as the by-product of distillation. However, more recently, both hydrosols and essential oils have become valued in equal parts for their therapeutic properties. Some plants are distilled solely for the hydrosol, even though they don't yield an essential oil, for example, cornflower (*Centaurea cyanus*).

Hydrosol is the common term that has been adopted in the United States to describe the final aromatic water product of distillation. However, there are many other terms that have been used, and are still used, to describe such a product. These include hydrolats (a term used in the UK and Europe), aromatic waters, floral waters (note, distilled waters are produced from more than just flowers), and essential waters.

Hydrosols are obtained via steam distillation from aromatic (and sometimes non-aromatic) plants which both yield, and do not yield, essential oils. During the distillation process, a certain percentage of water-soluble compounds are drawn into the steam (either from the essential oil molecules or independently, depending upon the plant) and are retained in the final water product.

Pure hydrosols hold therapeutic properties like essential oils, and they are often used in skin care. Hydrosols are less potent than essential oils because some of the more volatile chemical components found in essential oils are integrated through the volume of water in a hydrosol. They are extremely suitable for use with children and the elderly, due to their gentle nature.

Resins and Oleoresins

A resin is a solid or semi-solid in a natural or prepared format. Natural resins, such as gums, exude from the bark of a tree when it is cut. A product called a resinoid is prepared from the exudation of the tree sap. There is also a product called an oleoresin that is a prepared resin made from a mixture of essential oil and resin. Finally, a resin absolute is made from resin with the interjection of solvent.

Benzoin (*Styrax benzoin*) is an example of a resin extract that is prepared as a resin absolute (using solvents). Some plants may produce essential oils and oleoresins or resinoids, like myrrh (*Commiphora myrrha*).

Resins and their various product derivatives (such as resinoids and oleoresins) are complex areas that warrants further study. However, this chapter simply seeks to make you aware of such deviations from pure essential oils.

Absolutes and Concretes

Some plants produce a product called a concrete or an absolute. Again, concretes and absolutes are not essential oils, although some plant material can be used to produce both essential oils and concretes and absolutes. Due to methods of production, concretes and absolutes are not "pure" like essential oils and therefore do not hold the same therapeutic properties.

Concretes are prepared from plant material by the use of a hydrocarbon solvent to produce a waxy, solid substance. Absolutes are prepared from a concrete by alcohol extraction. Essential oils produced from solvent-extracted concretes and/or absolutes may retain a trace of the solvent in the end result.

Concretes and absolutes are predominately used for perfume products, but you will also find that some absolutes are used in aromatherapy practice, like jasmine (*Jasminum officinale*).

Carrier Oils

Carrier oils are the basis of therapeutic aromatherapy blends, particularly massage oils. Carrier oils help to blend together pure and volatile essential oils and consequently make a safer aromatic mix. Carrier oils have therapeutic properties in their own right, in addition to the essential oil properties in an aromatherapy blend.

In aromatherapy practice, the most common type of carrier oils are vegetable oils. However, base lotions, butters, balms, creams, and distilled water, are also "carriers" in aromatherapy. Vegetable oils used in aromatherapy are completely different to those used for cooking, and you should never substitute one for the other. Vegetable oils for aromatherapy use are usually fixed oils. A fixed oil is not volatile and therefore doesn't evaporate. A fixed oil is not soluble in alcohol and leaves a permanent oily mark on a piece of paper. As essential oils are volatile, they "dissolve" in carrier oils.

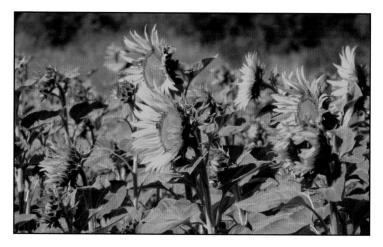

Photo copyright of Sharon Falsetto.

Cold-Pressed Vegetable Oils vs. Hot-Pressed Vegetable Oils

Ideally, you should choose a cold-pressed vegetable oil for aromatherapy use over a hot-pressed vegetable oil. Hot-pressed vegetable oils are subjected to a high level of heat in the extraction process and consequently do not retain the same therapeutic properties as a cold-pressed vegetable oil. In addition to basic vegetable oils, you will find macerated vegetable oils. These oils have been mixed with specific plant material to obtain additional therapeutic properties.

Cold-pressed carrier oils are obtained by pressing the seeds or nuts with a hydraulic press, which allows the oil to be "squeezed" out. If the nuts are hard, like those of safflower (*Carthamus tinctorius* L.), more force is needed to crush the nuts, and a machine called an expeller may be used. The carrier oil is then simply filtered out, to separate it from the crushed seeds and nuts.

Some of the more popular carrier vegetable oils include sweet almond (*Prunus dulcis*), jojoba (*Simmondsia chinensis*), sunflower (*Helianthus annuus*), coconut (*Cocos nucifera*), and argan (see below). Be aware that carrier oils can also be described as refined or unrefined, or organic or non-organic. An unrefined, or organic carrier oil, is usually superior in its properties and quality to a refined carrier oil.

A Note on Argan Oil

Perhaps one of the "hottest" carrier oils on the market at the moment is argan oil. Also known as Moroccan oil—because the oil is cold-pressed from the kernels of the Moroccan argan tree (*Argania spinosa*)—argan oil is expensive to buy because of its limited resources and the labor-intensive hours needed to produce a small quantity.

Argan oil is high in vitamin E. It is moisturizing and nourishing to the skin, especially for mature skin and wrinkles. Use it in a facial serum, in lotions and creams, as a massage oil, and in other moisturizing skin-care products like bath melts.

Make sure that you use cold-pressed argan oil that originates from Morocco—this is the only type of authentic argan oil available for aromatherapy use. Some aromatherapists prefer to use an alternate carrier oil because of the limited resources available for argan oil—and its high price—but it is a good, high-quality carrier oil if you are willing to use it.

5

Extraction of Essential Oils

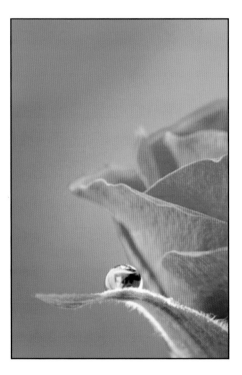

Essential oil production is increasingly becoming big business. There are a number of essential oil suppliers to choose from ranging from multi-level marketing (MLM) companies to the independent, family-operated business. Each company claims to offer the best quality essential oils, and it is a complex and time-consuming task for the consumer to assess fact from fiction.

Every reputable essential oil distributor supplies essential oils extracted by one of several methods, no matter where the essential oil began its journey. However, that journey from source (plant) to supplier—and ultimately the consumer—is long and will vary depending upon the plant source. Although techniques have improved over time for extracting essential oils, the basic method has remained the same.

Essential Oils in Plants

Plants go through a process called primary metabolism, which is vital to their continued existence. This process produces such products as sugar (obtained via photosynthesis) in order for the plant to live. In addition, plants go through secondary metabolism that produces products, among others, such as essential oils. It was originally thought that secondary metabolism products were of little importance to the plant, but this theory is starting to change as scientists study the role of essential oils in plant life.

Plants have to be able to deal with the world around them while literally being rooted to the spot. They both need to defend themselves against potential predators and attract pollinators for the continued evolution of their species. This has led to a development of tools for the plant, one of which is scent. Plants use scent to both "attract and defend," although it is worth remembering that not all plants are scented. In general, if a plant stores scent in the root, leaf, or bark, it is for defense purposes, whereas if a plant stores scent in the flower or fruit, it is for attracting purposes (i.e., as a pollination signal).

The scent in a plant is extracted and used for various aromatherapy purposes. The two main methods of essential oil (scent) extraction today are distillation and expression. Traditionally, enfleurage was a popular method for plant extraction but is a labor-intensive process that has more or less become obsolete in today's world. New methods, such as carbon dioxide extraction, are also emerging in the essential oil market.

Enfleurage

Enfleurage was traditionally used to make perfumes and was popular in Grasse, France, the traditional perfume capital of the world. Fragile flower blooms, such as jasmine, were particularly suited to this process.

The flowers were handpicked at sunrise, throughout the day, or at sunset, depending on the species of flower. Flowers were then left to macerate in oils and animal fat over a number of days. Different species of flowers required different time frames in which to extract the scent (essential oils) from the plant, and time frames ranged from days to weeks. Today, enfleurage has more or less been replaced by the process of solvent extraction.

Steam and Water Distillation

The majority of essential oils are extracted by water or steam distillation, but it is more common to use steam than water distillation. The difference between the two is that in water distillation the plant material is in direct contact with the water, whereas in steam distillation it is not. Steam distillation involves the use of high-pressure steam.

In steam distillation, plant material (such as leaves, flowers, twigs, or seeds) is placed in a huge vat and heated

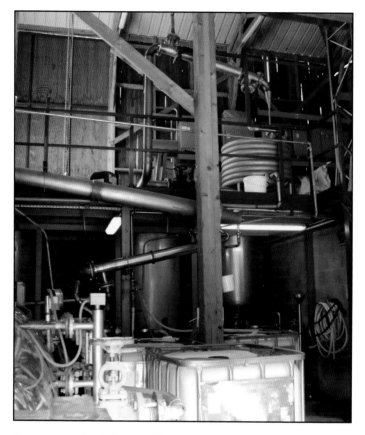

Photo copyright of Sharon Falsetto.

up. There are various sizes of vats, depending on the scale of the distiller's operation. As the plant material is heated up, essential oil molecules rise up and evaporate into the steam that is forced along a pipe. The pipe passes through another vat (this one is filled with cold water), and, as the steam cools, the essential oil molecules turn into liquid—the essential oil.

The essential oil molecules will either "sink" or "float" on the water, depending upon the type of plant from which the essential oil was extracted. The essential oil is then easily separated from the water (often used as a hydrosol) and drained off into a separate container.

It is worth noting that essential oils are not the exact chemical composition of the plant from which they were distilled. A number of factors will determine how closely an essential oil's chemical components will match the original plant's chemical components, including the method of distillation, the length of the distillation process (some plants take longer than others to distill), and the degree of heat used in the process.

Extraction by Expression

The term "expression" describes a method of squeezing or crushing the essential oil glands within the peel of citrus fruits to extract essential oil. Expression, or cold pressing, uses little to no heat in the extraction process, and it is usually reserved for citrus plants such as orange, lemon, and lime. Expressed essential oils are generally composed of the same chemical components that are found in the plant, due to method of extraction.

Citrus fruits store essential oils in the rind (or peel) of the fruit. They are extracted by a method of centrifugation, which essentially squeezes the juice (oil) out of the rind. Commercial equipment for extracting citrus oils may include pelatrice and sfumatrice. Essential oils extracted by this method also contain natural waxes and other non-soluble components. In addition, these types of essential oils may contain some chemical contaminants because of the chemicals used to spray fruit trees (unless they are grown organically).

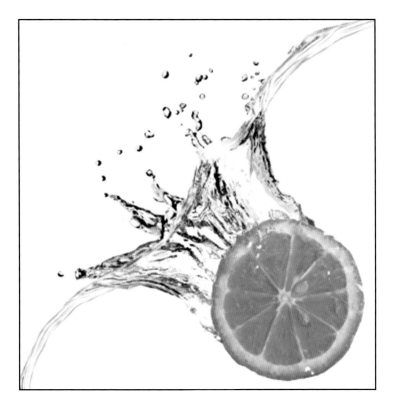

Cold-expressed essential oils do not have a very long shelf life, even if you are careful and store them under the right conditions (ideally in a cool, dark place in dark-colored, glass bottles). You also might find that citrus oils go cloudy after a while. In general, this does not affect the therapeutic properties of the oil. However, oxidization of an essential oil will affect the therapeutic properties. Grapefruit (*Citrus x paradisi*) essential oil has the shortest shelf life, and you should check that it has not gone rancid before using it.

Carbon Dioxide Extraction

Carbon dioxide extraction of essential oils is expensive and is not (as yet) as common as distillation. However, several essential oil distributors are now starting to offer a number of essential oils for sale that have been extracted by this method.

Carbon dioxide extraction involves the use of carbon dioxide at both high pressure and low temperatures in order to extract the essential oil from the plant. Essential oils produced through carbon dioxide extraction differ in chemical composition from essential oils produced through distillation.

Carbon dioxide extraction of essential oils is said to be more "pure" than the traditional method and closer to the original oil in the plant. There is no trace of carbon dioxide in the final essential oil produced. Although distillation of essential oils is also "pure," the chemical components of the final essential oil are slightly different in chemical composition from the original essential oil produced by the plant.

Research into the chemical composition of essential oils produced through carbon dioxide is not fully conclusive, given that it is a relatively new method in comparison to the distillation method for essential oil extraction. However, this may change in the future, depending upon the costs involved in such a method.

6

Quality of Essential Oils

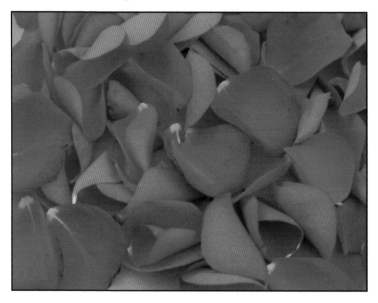

The quality (and price) of essential oils varies widely in the essential oil industry. Although small essential oil suppliers may have more expensive overhead costs than larger operators (who have the ability to produce more for less), the basic price of an essential oil should fall within a certain range typical for that particular oil. The quality of an essential oil might be affected by a number of factors, but the quality should still match that indicated in the standard test reports available for essential oils. If it does not, there is a good chance that the oil is of inferior quality or has been tampered with, commonly described by the term *adulteration* in the aromatherapy industry.

Adulteration of Essential Oils

A true essential oil is extracted from a plant, tree, or flower, either from its fruit, flowers, leaves, roots, or bark. The extraction of essential oils from different plants in different climates means that no two essential oils are exactly identical, even from the same species. Different batches of the same plant will often naturally produce a slight variation in chemical constituents of the essential oil.

However, a long and difficult extraction process equals high cost and labor in return for little quantity. These costs are passed onto the customer through a higher retail price in compensation for the effort (and money) put into producing such oils. Not all customers are willing to pay such a high price, leading to the producer coming up with inventive ways to lower cost. Unfortunately, this usually means a lower grade of essential oil and a preference for an increase in adulterated essential oils, particularly in the fragrance industry, where branding takes priority over authenticity.

The adulteration of an essential oil is relatively easy. An essential oil is usually adulterated via the introduction of an alcohol, a cheaper essential oil, or a synthetic product. This will both change the original quality (and properties) of the essential oil, and introduce other problems.

In true aromatherapy practice, authenticity and purity is of the utmost importance to the user. If you start altering the chemistry of the essential oil in any way, it will not hold the full therapeutic properties expected of the species from which it was extracted. Unpleasant side effects, such as skin irritations and nausea, may also occur. It is extremely important to preserve the synergy and wholeness of an essential oil for therapeutic use in true aromatherapy practice. Therefore, it is important to understand how and why adulteration takes place in essential oils and the tests carried out to ensure the quality of an essential oil.

Adulteration of Expensive Essential Oils

Tampering of an essential oil often occurs in species such as rose (*Rosa damascena*). Such plants emit only a minute quantity of essential oil at any one time with high labor costs. Rose is one of the most expensive essential oils on the market, yet many people are often unaware that they might not be purchasing true rose essential oil.

It takes approximately sixty thousand rose petals to produce just one ounce of oil. It is also estimated that there are over three hundred constituents that make up rose essential oil, making it relatively easy to substitute one or more of its chemical components. Geranium (*Pelargonium graveolens*) and palmarosa (*Cymbopogon martini*) are two of the most common substitutes for rose oil, although they both have independent therapeutic values, too. Be aware that rose absolute also exists and that there are distilled mixes of true rose essential oil with other true oils, such as rose geranium (not to be confused with *Pelargonium graveolens*).

Melissa (*Melissa officinalis*) is another essential oil that is frequently adulterated. Melissa oil is also called lemon balm, a reference to its fresh, lemony fragrance. Commercially produced melissa, and therefore not a true essential oil, often contains lemon (*Citrus limon*), lemongrass (*Cymbopogon citratus*), or citronella (*Cymbopogon nardus*) essential oils. The reason for the prohibitive cost of melissa oil is that it contains very little actual "oil" and is mainly made up of water. It requires a large quantity of plant material to produce a minute quantity of oil. Some producers choose to adulterate the oil to lower costs.

Fractionated Essential Oils

A fractionated oil is also a type of adulterated oil and is redistilled at a low pressure to isolate a number of chemical components. Fractionation results in a folded or terpeneless essential oil. Folded essential oils have a certain level of terpenes, determined by the processor, whereas terpeneless essential oils have the terpene component removed completely. Terpenes are considered of little or no value by some processors, although it completely unbalances, and therefore devalues, an oil for therapeutic use in aromatherapy.

Other Factors That Affect the Quality of an Essential Oil

Various factors naturally affect the quality of an essential oil, aside from tampering or adulteration. All essential oils are extracted from plants that have a country of origin. However, due to the cultivation of many plants worldwide, it is possible to find lavender (*Lavandula angustifolia*), for example, in many countries today, in addition to its native countries in the Mediterranean region. Quality and chemical makeup may vary widely in different types of essential oils grown outside of their country of origin. Other factors such as climate, soil quality, and the altitude at which a plant is grown can also affect the quality.

Although essential oils grown outside of their native country still contain therapeutic properties (provided that they are the true plant), check the chemical makeup to ensure that the oil contains the desired therapeutic properties. For example, some lavender essential oils contain a higher percentage of alcohols and/or esters, depending upon the country of origin and the altitude at which the plant was grown. A high altitude lavender contains more esters in its chemical components than a lower altitude lavender. And it is also worth remembering that "lavender" grown below an altitude of two thousand feet is not "true" lavender (*Lavandula angustifolia*); it is most likely the hybrid lavandin (*Lavandula x intermedia*). Some (disreputable) essential oil suppliers may label lavandin as lavender.

The quality of an essential oil is also affected by its method of extraction. As discussed previously, some producers might cut corners to maximize profits. The basic economic law of supply and demand can determine the quality of some essential oils. For example, frankincense (*Boswellia carteri*) is considered an endangered or threatened plant species. Demand for frankincense essential oil might soon start to exceed supply—and some suppliers might again start to cut corners (i.e., adulterate) lesser quality oils to meet demand. Several aromatherapists are making conscious decisions to use an alternative essential oil in place of an endangered or threatened species such as frankincense.

Quality Testing of Essential Oils

Quality testing of an essential oil ensures that a particular essential oil falls within the expected results for that oil, giving assurance that it has not been tampered or interfered with in any way. Essential oil quality tests attempt to determine the components of the essential oil and if any suspicious elements have been added or removed. The quality tests for essential oils include:

- Gas Liquid Chromatography (GLC)
- Mass Spectrometry (GC-MS)
- Optical Rotation
- Infrared Test
- Refractive Index

Gas Liquid Chromatography (GLC)

GLC separates the various components of the essential oil and produces a reading called a *chromatogram*. A chromatogram is essentially a "standard" reading to which subsequent essential oil readings can be compared and analyzed for differences.

In this particular test, the essential oil passes through a long tube (and various "stages" of gas and liquid within the tube) and, on evaporation at the other end, the trace of essential oil is recorded. Lighter essential oil molecules pass through the tube faster than heavier ones.

The results are compared to the "standardized" reading for that particular essential oil. It is only possible to compare essential oils generally to the "standard" reading as all pure essential oils are unique in their chemical makeup. However, certain chemical components should be present (or not present). Essential oil suppliers can usually supply you with such reports, although the information might not be presented in graph or pictorial form, depending upon supplier.

Below are two variations of standardized readings for anise star (*Illicum verum*) and amyris (*Amyris balsamiferia*) essential oils.

Both readings were provided by, and used with the kind permission of *Penny Price Aromatherapy*:

Certificate of Analysis – Amyris Oil
Species: *Amyris balsamifera*

Alpha-acoradiene	0.99%
<ar>-curcumene	1.34%
Beta-dihydroagarofuran	1.31%
Alpha-dihydroagarofuran	0.61%
7-epi-alpha-selinene	0.45%
Beta-sesquiphellandrene	1.48%
Delta-selinene	0.50%
Selina-3,7(11)diene	2.05%
Alpha-agarofuran	1.16%
Elemol	8.99%
(E)-nerolidol	0.36%
10-epi-gamma-eudesmol	7.51%
Gamma-eudesmol	7.98%
Beta-eudesmol	3.24%
Alpha-eudesmol	16.18%
Valerianol	17.04%
7-epi-alpha-eudesmol	7.21%
Drimenol	1.38%

Notes

The composition of the sample corresponds to that expected for the natural essential oil of *Amyris balsamifera*. Quality is exceptional with total sesquiterpene alcohols over 81%. Physical constants fall within acceptable ranges for the specified oil. No adulteration was detected.

Certificate of Analysis – Star Anise Oil
Species: *Illicium verum*

Linalool	0.60%
Alpha-terpineol	0.17 %
Carvone	0.01%
Beta-caryophyllene	0.50%
Beta-bisabolene	0.15 %
Alpha-copaene	0.05%
(Z)-Beta-farnesene	0.08%
Methyl chavicol	5.50%
(E)-Anethole	82.70%
Anisaldehyde	1.70%
Trans-anethole	0.15 %
Methyl-anisate	0.60%
P-Methoxyphenylacetone	0.20%
Cis-alpha-Bergamotene	0.10%
Trans-alpha-Bergamotene	0.25%
Foeniculin	5.10 %
Monoterpene hydrocarbons	3.00%
Cinnamyl alcohol	0.10 %

Notes
Antiviral and anti-flu in particular.

Gas Chromatography-Mass Spectrometry (GC-MS)

The GC-MS quality test is a more expensive test for essential oil quality. GC-MS is an advanced version of the Gas Liquid

Chromatography quality test. A reputable essential oil supplier should be able to provide the reports of either a GLC or GC-MS analysis of an essential oil to demonstrate the quality and purity of the essential oils that they are supplying.

The mass spectrometer is attached to the gas chromatograph, and the emerging essential oil molecules are hit with high energy electrons to separate them. GC-MS testing separates the individual components of the essential oil and allows identification of each chemical component by comparison to the molecular mass spectrum of the essential oil.

Optical Rotation, Infrared Testing, and Refractive Index

Optical rotation, infrared testing, and refractive index quality testing for essential oils are less common methods and more complex, scientific methods of essential oil quality testing. However, it is possible to see signs of adulteration with the infrared quality test if the person is an expert in his or her field. Refractive indexing produces consistent results for quality essential oil testing, and optical rotation testing produces results that allow the physical characteristics of an essential oil to be recognized.

Labeling of Essential Oils

A label says a lot about a product, yet, sometimes, you might not be aware of what is inside of the product if you don't understand the use of the terms. A reputable essential oil supplier should list the following information on the bottle of an essential oil (or in product supply lists):

- Country of origin
- Botanical name of the plant from which the essential oil was extracted
- Chemotype (if applicable)
- Organic (if applicable)
- Batch number
- "Use by" or distillation date
- Name of essential oil supplier
- Bottle size
- Contact details

In the United States, the term *therapeutic grade* is often used to describe the quality of an essential oil—this is not a legal term but a marketing term. Essential oil suppliers may use the term to describe their essential oils, indicating that the essential oils that they supply conform to "therapeutic grading" and are of superior quality than other suppliers that don't use the term. As any qualified aromatherapist will tell you, pure essential oils are, by their very nature, naturally "therapeutic grade."

Storage of Essential Oils

Storage of essential oils can affect quality too. Ideally, you should store essential oils in dark-colored, glass bottles and in a dark, cool place. Most essential oils are sold in amber-colored glass bottles. It is important to make sure that you don't store an essential oil in excess heat (and direct sunlight) as this can adversely affect its properties.

Citrus essential oils, particularly grapefruit (*Citrus x paradisi*), can oxidize quickly and lose their therapeutic properties, even when stored correctly. Citrus essential oils have a shorter shelf life than other essential oils.

Essential oils may last from one year (for example, grapefruit) to several years (for example, patchouli). Shelf life depends on the type of plant the essential oil was extracted from, storage, and several other factors.

Finding an Essential Oil Supplier

With a myriad of essential oil suppliers to choose from, it is difficult to know where to start when looking to find a reputable one. If you add in all the difficulties in ascertaining the quality of essential oil, how do you separate fact from fiction?

It is important to learn as much as you can about an essential oil, its typical behavior, appearance, and aroma before setting out on your search. If you know what to look for you will be more adequately equipped to assess the reliability and reputation of an essential oil supplier. Reputable essential oil suppliers have a good working relationship with and knowledge of the growers and farmers of the plants that produce their essential oils. They are also knowledgeable about individual essential oils and the variations available, essential oil testing, and all of the factors discussed in this chapter. However, recommendations of an essential oil supplier from a trusted source are probably still of the highest value.

7

Basic Chemistry of Essential Oils

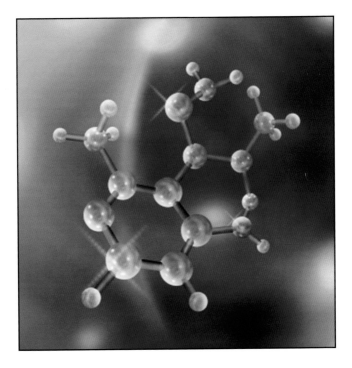

An essential oil is chemically composed of various components. The chemistry is complex, but a basic understanding
of the individual components is helpful to the beginner in

aromatherapy to help distinguish a true essential oil from a fake essential oil. In addition, it will help you to understand how the combination of various components contributes to the therapeutic properties of an oil. Essential oils hold many different chemical combinations. The proportion of each individual chemical component dictates, in general, the therapeutic properties of it.

Essential oils contain several major chemical components as discussed in this chapter, and the percentage of one particular component may dominate or change how another component acts within that essential oil. Essential oil molecules are made up of carbon, oxygen, and hydrogen atoms. Although this subject area requires further study for serious aromatherapists, in simple terms, an essential oil holds a combination of chemical molecules, formed from various versions of these atoms. The chemical components are listed from least to most volatile, following the description of terpenes. Terpenes make up the largest group of chemical components in essential oils and are present in most essential oils.

Terpenes

Terpene names usually end in -ene. The molecules that make up terpenes are light. You will find that many of the top note essential oils contain a high percentage of terpenes. Terpenes are antiseptic and often oxidize into alcohols over time (by combining with oxygen).

Terpenes are made up of isoprene units that are, essentially, one of the two main building blocks of essential oils; the other building block is the aromatic ring, a subject area that warrants further study for serious aromatherapists. Each isoprene unit contains five carbon atoms. The chemistry is more complex than is described here but, simply put, the type of terpene is defined by the number of isoprene units it holds. These can be subdivided as follows:

- Monoterpenes—hold two isoprene units. Examples include limonene, pinene, and camphene. Monoterpenes may be stimulating and irritating to the skin, if used in large quantities.
- Sesquiterpenes—hold three isoprene units. Examples include chamazulene, caryophyllene, and bisabolene. Sesquiterpenes are heavier than monoterpenes (both in scent and chemical components).
- Diterpenes—hold four isoprene units. Diterpenes are rare in essential oils.

Alcohols

An alcohol is formed in an essential oil from a complex combination of hydrogen and oxygen atoms. The name of the alcohol usually ends in -ol. Alcohols in an essential oil are categorized as monoterpenols, sesquiterpenols, and diterpenols. Monoterpenol alcohols are the least reactive, in terms of safety. An example of an alcohol component is linalool.

In therapeutic terms, alcohols are stimulating, antiviral, bactericidal, anti-infectious, and a tonic. In general, essential oils that are mainly composed of alcohols are nontoxic, nonirritant, and safe to use with children and older people.

Examples of essential oils with a high percentage of alcohol components include lavender (*Lavandula angustifolia*), geranium (*Pelargonium graveolens*), and rose (*Rosa damascena*).

Esters

Ester names usually end in the suffix *-ate*. Esters are rare in essential oils on their own and are usually combined with acids. Therapeutically, esters are anti-inflammatory, calming, balancing, useful in skin care, antifungal, nontoxic, and gentle to use. An example of an ester component is linaly acetate.

Examples of essential oils that contain a high percentage of esters include lavender (*Lavandula angustifolia*), clary sage (*Salvia sclarea*), and jasmine (*Jasminum officinale*).

Phenols

Phenols are similar to alcohols in essential oils but are stronger in their actions. Confusingly, phenol names also end in *-ol* so it is important to identify the individual chemical component and know if it is an alcohol or a phenol. For example, linalool is an alcohol component, whereas eugenol is a phenol component. There are more common alcohol components in essential oils than phenol components. Phenols may also appear as phenolic ethers in essential oils, for example, methyl chavicol. These types of components are more complex in structure than phenols and might be more neuro-toxic—but they have similar therapeutic properties.

The therapeutic properties of phenols are antiseptic, anti-bactericidal, anti-inflammatory, and stimulating. However, individual phenol components may or may not have some or all of these properties. Phenols are skin irritants if used in large quantities.

Examples of essential oils that contain a high percentage of phenol components include sweet fennel (*Foeniculum vulgare*), clove bud (*Syzygium aromaticum*), and cinnamon leaf (*Cinnamomum zeylanicum*).

Aldehydes

Aldehydes are commonly used in perfumery because they have a strong fragrance. The names of aldehyde components usually end in *-al*. Aldehydes should be treated with the same caution as ketones (see below) in aromatherapy use, although they are not as toxic as ketone components. An example of an aldehyde component is citral.

Aldehydes are anti-infectious, a tonic, anti-inflammatory, and calming when used therapeutically. Aldehydes may cause irritation and sensitization in some people.

Examples of essential oils that contain a high percentage of aldehyde components include melissa (*Melissa officinalis*), lemongrass (*Cymbopogon citratus*), and lemon-scented eucalyptus (*Eucalyptus citriodora*).

Ketones

Ketone components are often more hazardous and volatile than other chemical components in essential oils, but this does not mean that they should be avoided in their entirety. Not all ketone components are hazardous. In addition, a process known as quenching (when the presence of one component lessens the effects of another component) can often override the unwanted side effects of the more hazardous oil. However, it is necessary to treat the presence of ketones in essential oils with caution.

Ketone names usually end in *-one*, although there are exceptions to this general rule. An example of a ketone component is menthone.

Ketones, when used with care, are calming, sedative, digestive, analgesic, stimulant, expectorant, wound healing, and anti-
inflammatory in therapeutic value. Ketones vary, and some may
possess more of these properties than others, so it is advisable
to know the individual essential oil being used and the actual
ketones it possesses.

Essential oils that contain a high percentage of ketone
components include hyssop (*Hyssopus officinalis*), spearmint
(*Mentha spicata*), and common sage (*Salvia officinalis*).

Other Components

Other minor components in essential oils include oxides and
lactones. Oxides are rare in essential oils, with the exception
of *cineole*. Eucalyptol, 1,8-cineole, is an oxide that is found in
Eucalyptus Smithii, niaouli (*Melaleuca viridiflora*), and eucalyptus
blue gum (*Eucalyptus globulus*) in large quantities. It is mucolytic
(mucolytic agents help to unblock the airways) in its actions but
can be irritating to the skin if used in large quantities.

Lactones are present in most expressed oils but not in large
quantities. They have the same potential for neuro-toxicity as
ketones so should be used with care. Some essential oils also
contain coumarins and furocoumarins. Furocoumarins are
phototoxic in essential oils and therefore should be avoided
around sunlight and other forms of ultraviolet light. Furocoumarins are present in many expressed citrus essential oils, in
addition to a few other types of essential oils. Bergamot (*Citrus
bergamia*) essential oil possesses the furocoumarin, *bergapten*.

Essential Oils as a Whole

The chemical components of essential oils are not used individ-
ually, as broken down in this chapter, but with a combination of

one or more other chemical components in an oil. They are also often used in a blend of essential oils, combining the effects of all the components contained within those oils.

Combining both the individual chemical components found in essential oils and a number of different essential oils also produces varying therapeutic effects (known as a synergistic effect). If you understand the basic chemistry of the individual chemical components of essential oils and the general properties that they possess, you can learn to use essential oils both effectively and safely.

8

Species and Chemotypes

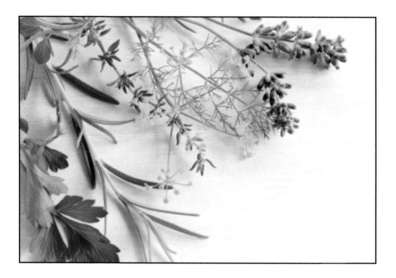

Essential oils are extracted from various plant species, and therefore it is important for beginners to aromatherapy to understand the definition of a plant species and how that plant species fits into the plant classification system, known as taxonomy. In addition to species, some plants produce chemotypes of essential oils. A chemotype is extracted from the same plant species but has varying chemical components.

Taxonomy

Taxonomy is the the classification of plants in botany. Taxonomy is important because many plants are commonly mistaken for others due to the use of common English names. For example, there are many varieties of rose. It is used as an essential oil in aromatherapy, yet the properties of a particular oil can vary, depending upon the variety of rose used. If you simply use the generic English name of rose, you can't distinguish if you are using *Rosa centifolia* or *Rosa damascena*.

Plant classification is not a simple process. A lot of plants are interrelated and resemble each other. The introduction of hybrids complicates matters further. However, according to the plant classification system, all plants are classified in an order, from the most basic to the most complex. A plant's botanical classification helps to describe its position in the plant kingdom and how it interacts with other plants.

Understanding Binomial Nomenclature

A Swedish botanist by the name of Carl Linneaus (1707–1778) invented the basis for a binomial nomenclature system in the eighteenth century. Under this system, a plant is given a binomial name, that is, a name in two parts. The binomial name consists of *genus* (generic) and *species* (specific). All names are in Latin, and the first part of the name, the genus, is a noun. The second part of the name, the species, is an adjective, which describes the genus.

For example, two different types of lavender can be described as follows: true lavender has a binomial name of *Lavandula angustifolia*, whereas spike lavender has a binomial name of *Lavandula latifolia*. *Lavandula* describes the genus, and the second part of the binomial name describes the species.

Thus, the binomial name of a plant describes the plant. The name can relate to the common name of the plant, describe the way it looks, indicate how the plant smells or tastes, any chemicals that may be present within the plant, or how the plant actually grows. It can also describe the plant's origin and can even be named after a prominent person. Some examples of the names of plants used in aromatherapy are described in the following table:

Common English Name	Family	Genus	Species*
Chamomile (Roman)	Asteraceae	Chamaemelum	(Chamaemelum) nobile
Ginger	Zingiberaceae	Zingiber	(Zingiber) officinale
Juniper	Cupressaceae	Juniperus	(Juniperus) communis
Lavender (true)	Lamiaceae	Lavandula	(Lavandula) angustifolia
Lemon	Rutaceae	Citrus	(Citrus) limon
Orange	Rutaceae	Citrus	(Citrus) sinensis
Rose	Rosaceae	Rosa	(Rosa) damascena

*Common usage usually combines both the genus and species name when identifying a plant species.

Aromatic Plant Families

Aromatic plants of the same plant family share not only similar physical characteristics but also similar therapeutic properties. Although it is possible to extract essential oils from over two hundred plants, not all of these oils are used in aromatherapy practice because of high toxicity levels in some plants.

The following table lists some of the common plant families used in aromatherapy, with an example of the essential oils

extracted from plants within that family and some of their shared
therapeutic properties:

Plant Family	Essential Oils	Therapeutic Properties
Abietaceae	Cedarwood (*Cedrus atlantica*), silver fir (*Abies alba*), pine (*Pinus sylvestris*)	Used for respiratory conditions
Apiaceae	Coriander (*Coriandrum sativum*), dill (*Anethum graveolens*), fennel (*Foeniculum vulgare*)	Balancing to digestive system
Asteraceae	Roman chamomile (*Chamaemelum nobile*), helichrysum (*Helichrysum angustifolium*), Moroccan chamomile (*Ormenis mixta*), German chamomile (*Chamomilla recutita*)	Soothing to skin and digestive system
Burseraceae	Frankincense (*Boswellia carteri*), myrrh (*Commiphora myrrha*)	Healing for wounds and scar tissue
Cupressaceae	Cypress (*Cupressus sempervirens*), juniper berry (*Juniperus communis*)	Used for stress and insomnia
Lamiaceae	Lavender (*Lavandula angustifolia*), patchouli (*Pogostemon cablin*), rosemary (*Rosmarinus officinalis*), peppermint (*Mentha piperita*)	Used for muscle pain, headaches, and as a nasal decongestant
Lauraceae	Cinnamon (*Cinnamomum zeylanicum*), rosewood (*Aniba rosaedora*), litsea (*Litsea cubea*)	Used for antiviral and anti-bactericidal properties

Plant Family	Essential Oils	Therapeutic Properties
Myrataceae	Tea tree (*Melaleuca alternifolia*), clove (*Syzigium aromaticum*), eucalyptus (*Eucalyptus smithii/ staigeriana*)	Used for respiratory conditions and as a strong antiseptic
Poaceae	Citronella (*Cymbopogon nardus*), palmarosa (*Cymbopogon martinii*)	Used for aches and pains, acne, and stimulating the circulation
Rutaceae	Bergamot (*Citrus bergamia*), lemon (*Citrus limon*), orange sweet (*Citrus sinensis*), neroli (*Citrus aurantium* var. *amara flos*)	Balancing to the digestive system and for skin conditions

Regional Aromatic Plant Species

It is common in today's aromatherapy world to find essential oils that have been extracted from regional plant species of common botanical genus. These essential oils are often described as "artisan" essential oils.

Essential oils extracted from regional plant species share common characteristics (and therapeutic properties) with their botanical cousins, but the chemical makeup of such an essential oil might vary slightly from components in the common genus. In addition, there is often little (or no) conclusive evidence to "prove" the therapeutic properties of regional essential oils in comparison to the more general plant species because such oils haven't been in popular use for a great length of time. There is also little information on any known contraindications for using the oil.

A reputable essential oil supplier who sells regional or artisan essential oils should be able to provide you with a GLC or GC-MS

data analysis to help you to determine the major chemical components of the essential oil, in comparison to the usual GC-MS data
analysis of the essential oil for that species. For example, compare
(common) cypress (*Cupressus sempervirens*) with a regional variation such as Arizona cypress (*Cupressus arizonica*), and make your
own assessment of the oil based on general therapeutic properties
known for the individual chemical components.

However, as some popular plant species become endangered or threatened due to popular use, regional essential oils
will probably start to increase in popularity. In addition, some
regional plants may emit essential oils not commonly used in
aromatherapy practice and lead to further research into these
particular essential oils.

Essential Oil Chemotypes

An essential oil chemotype is derived from a plant that has the
same visual appearance and characteristics, but it is chemically
composed of differing components. An essential oil chemotype has different therapeutic properties due to the presence of
different chemical components. For example, one chemotype may
have a higher content of alcohols compared to another chemotype
that may have a high content of phenols. Chemotypes are present
in both wild and cultivated plants.

Plant species produce different chemotypes for various
reasons. Factors that may affect the production of essential oil
chemotypes include:

- Climate
- Growing elevation of a plant
- Growing conditions of a plant
- Wild plant species may naturally cross-pollinate
- Other environmental factors

Identifying Essential Oil Chemotypes

To understand how essential oil chemotypes are identified, the following example of rosemary (*Rosmarinus officinalis*) is used. Rosemary has three common chemotypes that are used in aromatherapy. The abbreviation *ct.* is used following the binomial name of the plant to identify the type of chemotype of the essential oil. Therefore, rosemary essential oil can be described in one of the three following ways:

- *Rosmarinus officinalis* ct. camphor—high in camphor
- *Rosemarinus officinalis* ct. cineole—high in 1,8-cineole
- *Rosmarinus officinalis* ct. verbenone—high in verbenone

The therapeutic properties of each type of chemotype may vary, depending upon the essential oil. Examples of other essential oil chemotypes include (note, this list is not exhaustive):

- Basil (*Ocimum basilicum*)—ct. eugenol, ct. linalool
- Sage (*Salvia officinalis*)—ct. cineole, ct. thujone
- Thyme (*Thymus vulgaris*)—ct. thymol, ct. linalool, ct. carvacrol

There are also various other plants that can be used to distill chemotypes.

An essential oil supplier may or may not identify the chemotype of the essential oil on the label. However, common chemotypes, such as rosemary and thyme, are usually identified. Not all plants produce an essential oil chemotype, but if you are aware of the common plants that do, you will be able to choose the right type of essential oil for your purpose.

9

Endangered Essential Oils

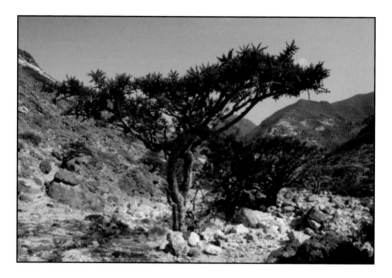

As aromatherapy grows in popularity, so does the use of essential oils. The demand for essential oils increases the need for plants to extract these oils from, and, although many plants are cultivated specifically for essential oil distribution, there are some plant species that have already become threatened or endangered by the increasing essential oil industry. In addition, species such as sandalwood (*Santalum album*) do not reach maturity until thirty years of age, meaning that it can take a long time to replace any trees that are harvested and exhausted for their essential oil use.

Several essential oils are extracted from plant species that are either under threat of extinction or classed as an endangered species. Awareness about this growing problem has prompted some growers (and users of essential oils) to cultivate alternative species.

Whether you choose to continue to use endangered or threatened plant species for essential oil use, or find an alternative substitute, it is helpful to have an understanding of the problem in order to make an informed decision.

The IUCN Red List of Threatened Species

The International Union for Conservation of Nature (IUCN) is an organization that was initially set up to assess the conservation status of plant and animal species in the world, highlighting those species that are threatened with extinction, and promote the cause for their conservation.

The IUCN was established in October 1948 as the International Union for the Protection of Nature (IUPN). In 1956, the organization changed its name to the International Union for the Conservation of Nature (IUCN). IUCN was the world's first global environmental organization. Today, it is the largest professional global conservation network. The primary mission of the IUCN is to encourage and to help the world's societies to conserve nature and the wide range of both animal and plant species. It also makes sure that natural resources are ecologically sustainable.

The IUCN produces a document called the Red List of Threatened Species. This list is defined as "the world's most comprehensive inventory of the global conservation status of plants, animals, and fungi and the most authoritative guide to the status of biological diversity" (www.IUCN.org).

The IUCN lists nine categories in the Red List of Endangered Species:

- Extinct
- Extinct in the wild
- Critically endangered
- Endangered
- Vulnerable
- Near threatened
- Least concern
- Data deficient
- Not evaluated

Species are categorized according to an assessment by scientists, based on factors such as rate of decline, size of population, and area of distribution.

Threatened and Endangered Plant Species
A threatened species is "a species of (animal or) plant that is rare and may become an endangered species in the near future" (*Webster's* 2009). An endangered species is "a species of (animal or) plant in danger of becoming extinct" (*Webster's* 2009).

Threatened and Endangered Essential Oils
There are several common essential oils in use that are extracted from threatened or endangered plant species. According to the National Association for Holistic Aromatherapy (NAHA), frankincense (*Boswellia carteri*), sandalwood (*Santalum album*), agarwood (examples: *Aquilaria malaccensis*, *Aquilaria agallocha*), and rosewood (*Aniba rosaeodora*) are threatened or endangered. The plants from which these particular essential oils are extracted

from might be in danger of disappearing from Earth completely if the industry continues to use them to excess. Note, however, that this is an ongoing issue, and situations change all the time, depending upon various factors. Check up-to-date resources for the latest available information. Alternate essential oils for frankincense and sandalwood are suggested in *Part Three*.

If you decide to use an alternate essential oil in preference to one of those that is considered either threatened or endangered, you need to check the chemical constituents of the essential oil and therapeutic properties to establish whether the proposed alternative will perform the same functions. In addition, if you are choosing an essential oil simply for its fragrance, you will need to experiment with the type of base product you intend to use it with; for example, certain types of candle wax do not always retain the expected aroma of the essential oil. However, it is usually preferable to use an alternative essential oil over a synthetic substitute in aromatherapy because a synthetic substitute has no therapeutic properties and does not mimic the true scent of an essential oil.

10

Home Distillation of Essential Oils

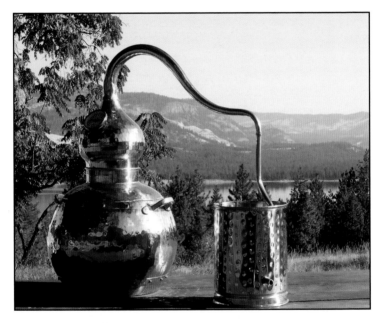

Photo copyright of Ann Harman.

The distillation of essential oils is a complex process. Although it is possible to distill your own essential oils at home, the process is often time consuming with little oil extracted, depending on the type of plant you choose to distill. However, the quality of the essential oil will probably be superior when compared to some commercial essential oils—and you will know exactly what went into (or not into) the distillation of it.

Note that the information contained in this chapter refers to personal use of essential oils. If you intend to sell your distillate, there is a series of tests, and legislation to follow, depending upon various factors.

Plant Quantity and Other Variables

If you use the right type of plant material and know the expected amounts of production, it is possible to produce high quality, therapeutic essential oils for your personal needs. A major factor in deciding if you have the resources to distill your own essential oils at home is the quantity of plant required to distill a specific amount of essential oil. The following examples give you an idea of what to expect if you distill the plants of lavender or rose:

- Lavender (*Lavandula angustifolia*)—it takes one hundred and fifty pounds to produce one pound of lavender essential oil. One acre of land produces between twelve and twenty pounds of lavender essential oil (www.auracacia.com).
- Rose (*Rosa damascena*)—it takes two hundred and fifty pounds to produce one ounce of rose essential oil (www.britannica.com).

Bear in mind that these amounts are approximations only and can vary due to a number of other factors including:

- Growing season
- Quality of original plant material (organic/wild/cultivated/sprayed with chemicals)

- Climate and weather patterns
- Quality of soil
- Age of plants

Plant Your Own Aromatherapy Garden

In addition to distilling plant material to produce your own essential oils, you can also plant your own aromatherapy garden to experience the scent of individual plants. This is not a new concept. Fragrant and medicinal plants were prominent in medieval monastery cloister gardens. The cloister garden was an enclosed, green space within the monastery, based on the style of Roman villa gardens. It provided a place of relaxation among the aromatic plants. In addition, medieval monasteries were home to herb gardens, which were split into a physics garden full of healing herbs and plants, and a kitchen garden, where herbs were grown for use in culinary dishes.

You don't need a large space to grow several types of aromatherapy plants in your own garden. Fragrant herbs and plants such as lavender, rosemary, and geranium can be grown on a small patio with the right growing conditions. If you only have a window box, consider a fragrant variety of herbs, such as thyme and peppermint.

Essential Oils, Infused Oils, and Flower Essences

If you are considering distilling your own essential oils, it is important to distinguish the difference between essential oils and infused oils. Essential oils are distilled directly from the plant (using the methods discussed in chapter 5), whereas infused oils involve the use of a carrier oil base. In addition, essential oils are often mistakenly referred to as *essences*, leading to further confusion with actual flower essences. Flower essences are collected through a combination of water and sunlight and are not distilled like true essential oils.

The therapeutic properties of each of these types of oils (and chemical makeup of the oil) will, therefore, vary.

Home Distillation Kits

Photo copyright of Ann Harman.

The easiest way to make your own essential oils at home is by using an essential oil distillation kit. There are several kits now on the market specifically designed for distilling at home. Although these kits might involve a hefty sum of money as an initial investment, they do contain all of the equipment needed to get you started in making your own oils. Purchase a kit from a reputable essential oil distiller, rather than a mainstream manufacturer. An experienced distiller will be able to offer you advice on using the kit from their own personal knowledge.

In addition to using a home distillation kit for essential oils, you can also distill hydrosols in a still. Stills are usually available in stainless steel or copper. Ann Harman, a certified organic farmer located in Washington state, has been distilling hydrosols for over fifteen years and believes that copper stills are better for the distillation of hydrosols. She is in the process of trying to prove that the copper in copper stills remains in the distillate to help with microbial contamination. She presented her early findings of this process at the Botanica conference in Dublin, Ireland in 2012.

How to Make an Infused Oil

If you want to make an infused oil as opposed to a true essential oil, you can do so with minimum investment. All you need to get started are a few basic items:

- A jar in which to place your fresh plant material—a Mason jar is ideal.
- Vegetable carrier oil—you will need to choose a suitable vegetable carrier oil base in which to diffuse your plant material.
- A strainer or a sieve—at the end of the diffusion, you will need to separate your plant material from your oil using a strainer or a sieve (a regular kitchen sieve will work).
- Sunshine

Follow these simple instructions to make an infused oil:

- Collect fresh plant material or dried herbs and place them inside a jar.
- Fill the jar with enough oil to completely cover the plant material.
- Leave the jar in sunshine for one to two weeks. A sunny window ledge is a good place to leave your infusion to work.
- Add more plant material (to fill up the jar as necessary) and shake up the jar intermittently.
- After one to two weeks, separate the plant material from the oil with the sieve or strainer.

If your infusion is successful, your oil should have a fragrant aroma—and it will possess the therapeutic properties of the plant. In some cases, you might want to leave the plant material soaking for a longer period of time in order to diffuse more effectively. In addition, you can make infused oils from plants or herbs that are not distilled for essential oils, for example, St. John's wort and calendula.

More Information on Flower Essences

Flower essences became popular through the work of Dr. Edward Bach (1886–1936), an English physician who carried out extensive research on the therapeutic benefits of essences. Other types of flower essences include Australian Bush Flower Essences.

Flower essences correspond to a *virtue*, or emotional imbalance, in the body that causes dis-harmonization. A suitable flower essence is chosen to address and rebalance the body. Although essences are referred to in general as flower essences, essences do include trees, too, like elm, honeysuckle, heather, and oak. These are plant species that are not commonly used for essential oil distillation (although honeysuckle produces a minute quantity of essential oil, which is used in perfumery).

Plant material is collected from the plant, placed in a bowl of water, and allowed to infuse the natural elements of the sun (or other heat source) and air. Once the plants have been infused for a period of time, the water infusion is bottled and stored, ready for use. Flower essences also contain alcohol (usually brandy) as a natural preservative for the infusion. Flower essences are said to contain the vibration, or energy, of the plant, which is used to heal the imbalances in the body.

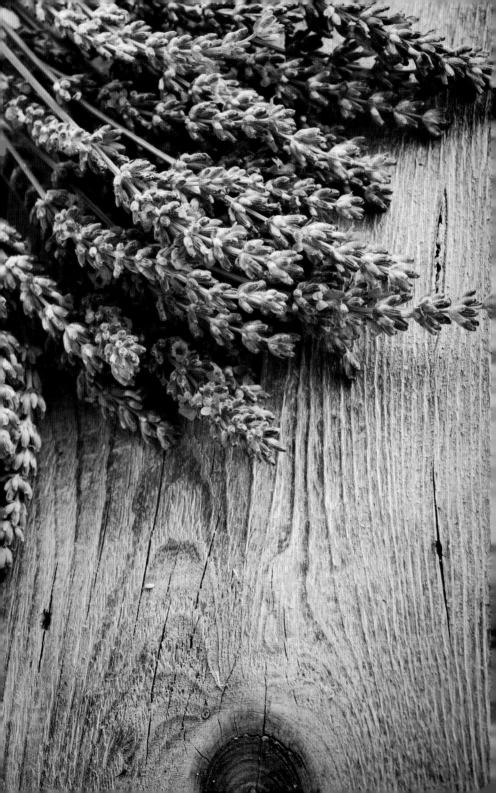

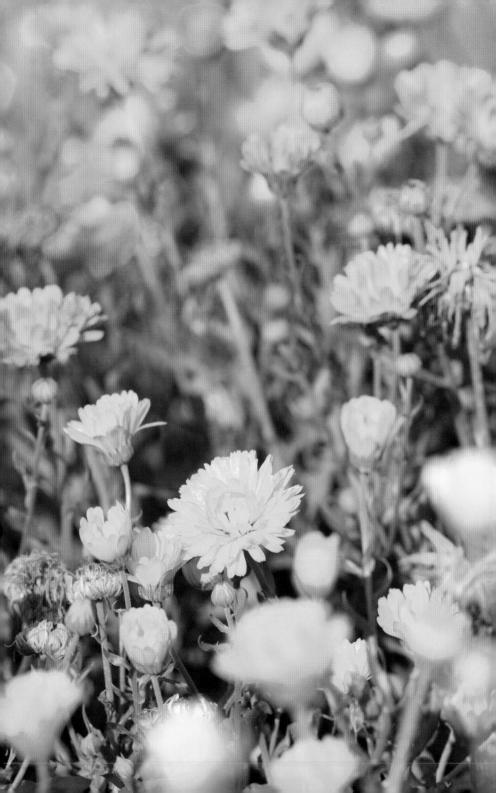

Part Two

Using Essential Oils

11

Cautions and Tips for Using Essential Oils

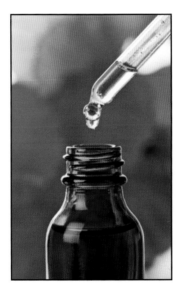

An essential oil may, or may not, have specific cautions for use, depending on the chemical components from which it is made. The essential oils that are profiled in this book are listed in *Part Three*, along with any specific cautions for using them. However, in addition to these specific cautions, there are also general guidelines to keep in mind.

Using Essential Oils in Pregnancy

Pregnancy is a time when essential oils should be treated with caution, particularly during the first trimester of pregnancy. Essential oils for pregnancy are discussed in further detail in chapter 16. However, examples of essential oils that are often contraindicated for use in pregnancy include cinnamon (*Cinnamomum zeylanicum*), clove (*Syzygium aromaticum*), hyssop (*Hyssopus officinalis*), peppermint (*Mentha piperita*), rosemary (*Rosmarinus officinalis*), and sage (*Salvia officinalis*).

Essential oils are thought to be capable of crossing the placental barrier because of their molecular weight and high negative charge (Price and Price, 2002). Although the effects of how essential oils might affect both mother and baby are not proven scientifically, caution is usually advised for use of essential oils in the first trimester of pregnancy when there is a higher risk of miscarriage.

Always use a lower dilution of essential oils in pregnancy. In addition, it is essential to liaise with a midwife who has experience with using essential oils with pregnant women. Some aromatherapists have specialized training in using essential oils in pregnancy, but little is yet proven about how essential oils may affect pregnant women. Several essential oils are contraindicated for use by one source and not another, so it is important to understand as much as you can about the individual chemical components that make up a specific essential oil and its possibility for contraindications for use. Finally, each pregnancy and health history is unique, and what might affect one woman, may not affect another, depending upon individual circumstances.

Using Essential Oils with Babies and Children

As discussed in chapter 17, essential oils are great for using with babies and children because they are usually very receptive to the idea. However, specific essential oils that you should avoid with babies and children are also discussed in chapter 17, and it is important to remember these cautions. In addition, remember to use a lower dosage of essential oils for babies and children, too. Consult with a qualified nurse or health practitioner who has training in the use of essential oils for babies and children for further advice, or ask a certified aromatherapist who has taken specific training in the area.

Using Essential Oils with Medical Conditions

Certain medical conditions are contraindicated for use of essential oils. Again, it is advisable to consult with your own health care practitioner on your individual health history and the potential risk for using essential oils. The following guidelines apply, in general, to those conditions listed, with an example of the essential oil to avoid in such circumstances (this list is not exhaustive and may include other essential oils):

- Allergies and sensitive skin—avoid the use of peppermint (*Mentha piperita*) essential oil and clove (*Syzygium aromaticum*) essential oil.
- Diabetes—use extra caution in the use of all essential oils.
- Epilepsy—avoid the use of rosemary (*Rosmarinus officinalis*) essential oil.
- High blood pressure—avoid the use of sage (*Salvia officialis*) essential oil.
- Low blood pressure—avoid the use of lavender (*Lavandula angustifolia*) essential oil.
- Migraine—avoid the use of rose (*Rosa damascena*) essential oil and lavender (*Lavandula angustifolia*) essential oil.

- Serious, recent illnesses—consult your health practitioner on individual circumstances.

Using Essential Oils with Other Treatments and Medication

Essential oils might interact with other treatments and medications, including both prescribed medication and over-the-counter medication. In addition, a complementary therapy treatment, in particular homeopathy, might be contraindicated with the use of essential oils because it may counteract the effectiveness of essential oil use. Know which medication or treatment you are using, and consult your health practitioner for further advice.

Using Essential Oils in the Sun or with Tanning Units

Some essential oils are described as phototoxic or photosensitive. Phototoxic essential oils react to sunlight, or ultraviolet light, which is used in tanning units. Most citrus essential oils are phototoxic, although it can depend upon their method of extraction. For example, expressed sweet orange (*Citrus sinensis*) essential oil is not phototoxic, but distilled sweet orange (*Citrus sinensis*) is. Bergamot (*Citrus bergamia*) essential oil is considered to be highly phototoxic because of the presence of bergapten in the essential oil. For this reason, some producers are now making bergapten-free bergamot essential oil. Other phototoxic essential oils include some non-citrus essential oils such as cumin (*Cuminum cyminum*), ginger (*Zingiber officinale*), and lovage (*Levisticum officinale*). Limit exposure to sunlight and other forms of ultraviolet light when using phototoxic essential oils to avoid excessive burning or skin sensitivities.

Other General Cautions for Use of Essential Oils

In addition to those cautions given in this chapter, and within the individual essential oil profiles, remember the following general cautions for using essential oils:

- Always dilute an essential oil in a carrier lotion, oil, or base, before applying it to the skin. In addition, do a small "patch" test before applying a blend to a wider area of skin.
- Avoid contact with the eyes.
- Avoid contact with mucous membranes, like the nose, eyes, and lips.
- Keep essential oil bottles out of reach of babies and children.
- Keep essential oil bottles out of reach of pets.
- Do not use essential oils internally without specialized training and the appropriate license to practice to do so in the country in which you live. In addition, some essential oils should never be used internally due to their toxicity.
- Discontinue use of essential oils if irritation or skin sensitivity occurs.
- Use in low concentration (or not at all) in pregnancy, with babies and children, with the elderly, and with those who have a serious illness.
- Use only pure essential oils to minimize the risks of potential negative or hazardous reactions.

- Keep essential oils away from heat, ignition sources, and flames; essential oils are flammable and are hazardous, under conducive conditions.
- The chemical components and therapeutic properties of an essential oil are not an exact duplication of the plant from which it was extracted.
- Educate yourself fully on the nature and use of an essential oil before using it.

Recommended Amounts for Essential Oils

The following chart indicates the general recommended amounts for using essential oils. It is intended as a guideline only, and you should remember to take into account personal health history, the type of essential oil used, the way in which an essential oil is used, and any contraindications for use.

The amounts in the following chart are based on use for a healthy adult and are based on personal, professional experience. Reduce or increase these amounts in proportion to size of the corresponding bottle, jar, or candle. In addition, reduce the amounts for babies and children, in pregnancy, with the elderly, and with serious illnesses.

ESSENTIAL OIL BLENDING CHART

PRODUCT	ESSENTIAL OIL DILUTION
Body Lotion/Cream/Butter (4 oz)	36–40 drops
Face Lotion/Cream/Butter (4 oz)	20–25 drops
Body Massage Oil (4 oz)	36–40 drops
Face Massage Oil (4 oz)	20–25 drops
Lip Balm (0.15 oz)	3–7 drops
Body Balm (0.15 oz)	5–8 drops

PRODUCT	ESSENTIAL OIL DILUTION
Bath Salts (4 oz)	40–50 drops
Sugar or Salt Scrub (4 oz)	20–30 drops
Personal Spray (4 oz) Room Spray (4 oz)	Up to 45 drops Up to 50 drops
Room Diffuser (Candle or Electric) (In addition, consult manufactur- er's instructions for use)	Up to 5 drops
Personal Inhaler (Standard Size)	10–15 drops
Body Compress (Average-sized Face Cloth)	5–10 drops
Tea Light Candles (0.5 oz)	Up to 20 drops (but varies according to blend)

General Blending Guidelines for Essential Oils

Success in blending essential oils comes through experience, depending on the product base and the essential oil used. However, the following general blending tips might help you to get started on successfully blending essential oils:

- Less is more—an optimum blend usually contains between one and three essential oils. Although some blends might contain up to five essential oils, the more essential oils that you blend together, the more they might begin to conflict with one another, in both scent and therapeutic properties.
- Top, middle, and base note—natural perfumers usually use a base note as a fixative for a blend and then mix in middle and top notes. Although it is not necessary to use a balance of top, middle, and base notes in a

therapeutic blend, it is something to consider when blending for scent.

- Synergy—a synergistic blend of essential oils is a blend that is greater than the sum of the individual essential oils. However, synergy also exists in a single essential oil, due to the various chemical components, and therefore it is important to use a pure, unadulterated essential oil in order to maintain this synergy.
- Quantity—base note essential oils are usually more powerful in fragrance and last longer than top note essential oils.
- Base medium—the base medium of your product will sometimes dictate an adjustment to the quantity of essential oil used. For example, a water-based spray usually requires more essential oil drops than a lotion base. In addition, reduce quantities for products used on the face in comparison to the rest of the body, due to sensitivity.

The Safety of Essential Oils

Essential oils are safe to use if you understand how, when, and where to use them. By following the contraindications for use and applying the knowledge and guidance of a professional, you can use essential oils in many different circumstances, without significant risk. Lack of knowledge and understanding leads to potential dangers and risks in using essential oils. Educate yourself fully before using essential oils to avoid these potential dangers.

12

How Essential Oils Work

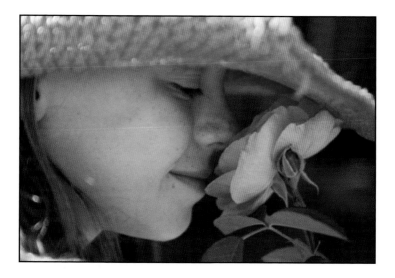

There is much debate over how essential oils work. Various scientific studies have been carried out over the years to either prove or disprove how essential oils access the body and affect our well-being. In addition, the term *aromatherapy* has been overused and adopted by many parts of commercial industry to the point that people may believe that synthetic aromas work in the same way as essential oils. Synthetic aromas (including fragrance oils) do *not* possess the therapeutic properties of essential oils and should not be used in the same ways as described in this chapter.

It is also important to make the distinction between essential oils and the use of plants and herbs as a medicine. Although plant medicine and use of plant oils date back thousands of years, these are not the same substances that we call essential oils today. The chemical makeup, and therefore the therapeutic properties, of essential oils may be different from those described in ancient texts.

There are several common theories within the aromatherapy profession as to how essential oils may work:

- Through inhalation
- Topically
- Internally

Despite the sometimes scarce scientific evidence of how essential oils work, many have been using essential oils for medicinal purposes for years. Often, it is difficult to carry out a scientific study without bias and with success, due to lack of funding, resources, and suitable participants. The interest in essential oils in recent years does, however, demonstrate the public's growing awareness of essential oils.

Inhalation of Essential Oils

Inhalation is accepted by most aromatherapists as the fastest and quickest way in which an aroma from an essential oil accesses the body. Scientific studies on this method of using essential oils is limited because an unbiased result is difficult to obtain, given that most participants in a study will be aware of the introduction of some type of aroma. It is difficult to administer some participants with a placebo and others with a real treatment with regard to smell.

However, some scientific studies do show that essential oils may have an effect through inhalation. For example, a study carried out with the use of lavender essential oil through inhalation on dementia patients appeared to show a reduction in agitation among them (van der Ploeg et al. 2010).

In addition, general science confirms that smell has a direct link to the brain. As you breathe in an aroma through your nose, the aroma passes through the respiratory system. Along the way, electrochemical messages are sent to the appropriate part of the brain, triggering the release of neuro-chemicals and allowing the brain to process different smells. These actions all occur at lightning speed.

Smells often act on both an emotional and physical level within the body. Your emotions are strongly intertwined with your physical well-being. The physical properties of an essential oil will usually work despite a person's negative reaction to an oil on a physical level, but the emotional effects of an essential oil will depend heavily on a person's openness to it, in particular to scent.

As discussed above, aromas enter the body physically through inhalation, by way of the nose. Inhalation of essential oils is believed to act on an emotional level due to the direct link to the brain. A system in the brain, called the limbic system, is strongly believed to link to emotions. Hair cells (receptors) respond to smells inhaled by the nose and transmit this information to the olfactory bulb via mitral cells. The olfactory tract transmits this information to parts of the limbic system, such as the hippocampus, amygdala, and the hypothalamus. The limbic system is strongly associated with memory. Therefore, certain smells trigger certain memories.

Many people use essential oils for emotional issues such as stress, anxiety, and depression for the "feel good" factor that certain essential oils invoke through stimulation of the limbic system. Although the process of how such aromas work is more complex than that described above, it does show that aromas have a significant effect on both the physical and emotional body.

Methods of inhalation of essential oils include candles, sprays, tissues, baths, diffusers, and vaporizers. These methods are discussed in greater detail in chapter 13.

Topical Application of Essential Oils

The topical application of essential oils is usually through application to the skin. Many argue that it is not possible for essential oils to access the bloodstream via the skin because it is perceived as an impermeable organ. However, if you think about how ancient Egyptian women used oils as beauty cosmetics, people have been using the practice for thousands of years without scientific evidence to justify the reasons for doing so.

Price and Price in *Aromatherapy for Health Professionals* cite the study of Jäger et al. (1992) that shows that the use of lavender essential oil applied in a base oil was absorbed into the bloodstream. Although different chemicals are absorbed in different quantities and at various rates by the body, it appears that it is possible that certain chemical compounds can penetrate the skin. For example, the smaller, lighter molecules of top note essential oils are absorbed more quickly into the skin than larger, heavier, base note essential oils. Absorption rates may also be affected by heat, massage, condition of the skin, and breathing rate.

Methods of topical application of essential oils include massage, baths, compresses, and sprays. These methods are discussed in greater detail in chapter 13.

Internal Use of Essential Oils

The internal use of essential oils is perhaps the most hotly contested and discussed method of application of essential oils. Ingestion of essential oils through the mouth, rectum, and vagina, is an area of study that should be understood in great detail before any attempts. The use of essential oils in this way is often called aromatic medicine and should only be used by those with a detailed understanding of how to do it safely. There are various myths and beliefs (some of which are dangerous) of how to administer essential oils internally.

It is *extremely* important to have knowledge of the chemical components of essential oils and the known contraindications before using them internally. You should also know the proper amounts to use (usually a minute quantity). There is strong potential for toxicity if not used correctly. Remember to dilute in a carrier (oil, water, etc.), too. In addition, some essential oils should never be used in this way simply because of their toxic makeup. Finally, it is of the utmost importance that you use true essential oils and not adulterated essential oils.

It is also worth noting that the use of essential oils when used this way is regarded as a branch of medicine in some countries— and it is illegal to carry out such a practice professionally without a license. Consider contraindications for use, such as pregnancy and with babies and children, where care is paramount. *Consult a qualified professional who is trained in aromatic medicine before attempting to use essential oils in this way.* Education is the key to the internal use of essential oils safely and should not be advocated by untrained or unlicensed professionals.

A Note on How Carrier Oils Work

As discussed in chapter 4, carrier oils are one of the main mediums used to apply essential oils topically. Carrier oils access the body in much the same way as essential oils do. Until the end of the nineteenth century, it was believed that the skin could not absorb soluble solutions such as carrier oils (studies such as Fleischer's [1877] concluded this). However, various studies in the twentieth century (including that of Valette and Sorbin [1963]) have concluded that carrier oils can be absorbed by the skin and thus be therapeutic to the body.

How Essential Oils Access the Body

Although scientific studies are often limited in their conclusions on the effectiveness of essential oils, this does not mean that essential oils don't work. Essential oils have been used for many years for various conditions by aromatherapists. In addition, new research emerges all the time on how aromatherapy works, so check the latest scientific studies for new information. Many studies are now available online via university and scientific journal websites.

13

Ways to Use Essential Oils

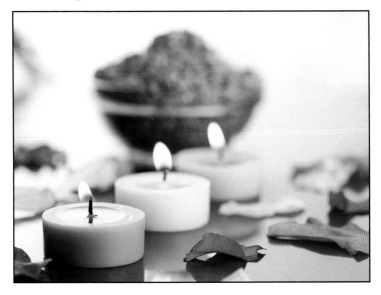

There are many different ways in which you can use essential oils, but it is important to know how to practice each method safely. Certified aromatherapists are trained with regard to both the type and quantity of each essential oil to use, depending upon the method of administration and any contraindications that might prevent a particular essential oil from being used safely.

This chapter discusses the various methods for using essential oils. General guidelines for the amounts to use are given in chapter 11.

Inhalation

Inhalation is one of the easiest ways to use essential oils. The following methods are recommended.

Candles

It is important to note that not all aromatherapy candles are created equal, and you should check the ingredients and specifics of each candle before using it. Look at the type of wax it is made with, the type of wick used, and the ingredients used to scent it. If you purchase an aromatherapy candle from a commercial chain, it is probably not a true aromatherapy candle but a paraffin-based candle, with a synthetic fragrance. These types of candles typically cost a few dollars but may present a wide range of health risks, such as asthma, breathing difficulties, and even cancer.

A true aromatherapy candle is made with pure essential oils and a natural base of wax (made of beeswax or soy). Some suppliers also go to great lengths to research the right type of wick for a particular candle, such as a paper-core or cotton wick. It is simple to make your own aromatherapy candles with soy wax or beeswax. The easiest way to start is to purchase a candle-making kit from a candle-making supplier and add in your chosen essential oils.

Many small businesses who make true aromatherapy candles will be happy to "educate" you about aromatherapy candles if you ask them. The price will typically be higher than a store-bought candle, but it will contain true aromatherapy ingredients.

Sprays

It is relatively easy to make your own spray with essential oils. All you need are the following products:

- An empty spray bottle
- Chosen essential oils
- Distilled water

Simply fill the empty spray bottle with distilled water, add in essential oils, and shake the bottle to mix. Oil and water do not typically gel together but if you shake the bottle vigorously, it should be sufficient to emit the aroma. You can also add a dispersing agent, such as a natural Solubol.

You can use aromatherapy sprays to mist a room, yourself, or your car. For best results, use immediately, store away from sunlight, and use within a couple of weeks of making the product.

Aromatherapy Diffusers and Vaporizers

There are now a couple of varieties of aromatherapy diffusers and vaporizers on the market, in addition to the traditional candlelit diffuser. The terms *diffuser* and *vaporizer* are used interchangeably, often to describe the same, or similar, product. Technically, vaporizers push the lightest essential oil molecules out first, whereas diffusers push all of the essential oil molecules out at the same time (Price and Price 2012).

Candle diffusers require the addition of a few drops of essential oil to water, which are placed in a ceramic tray on top of the diffuser. Put a lit candle underneath the tray (usually a tealight candle) to allow the water to heat up and diffuse the essential oils into the air. Do not leave the diffuser unattended. You should also make sure that sufficient water is added to the tray on top of the diffuser because the essential oil can "burn out."

Electric aromatherapy diffusers are considered the safest type of aromatherapy diffuser. They usually have a glass container to hold the oils. The diffuser pushes the different-sized essential oil molecules out at the same time. Electric aromatherapy diffusers have become more economical and environmentally friendly over time. Some types of electric diffusers now have silver ion sterilization technology, which increases resistance to mold and corrosion while deodorizing and sterilizing.

Electric nebulizing aromatherapy diffusers force air into the essential oils through an air pump. When the essential oil molecules are released into the air through means of a glass "nebulizer," they are micro-sized. The result is a therapeutic blend of essential oils that is dispersed into the air and readily breathed in. Nebulizing aromatherapy diffusers are popular for respiratory conditions.

You can also purchase a plug-in aromatherapy diffuser for your car. The diffuser is powered by the cigarette lighter outlet or cell phone charger. It contains a small pad onto which you can add a few drops of essential oils. The heat from the outlet disperses the aroma around the vehicle.

There are always new essential oil diffusers coming onto the market, so check out the latest, and decide which is best for you. Other ways of diffusing essential oils include the use of terracotta and sandstone diffusers (various shapes, sizes, and styles), fan diffusers (often portable), and lamp ring diffusers. Lamp ring diffusers are often popular because of their relatively inexpensive cost. They are shaped like a ring, made of terracotta or brass, and have a grooved dip where the essential oil is placed. The heat from the bulb allows for the dispersal of the oil.

It is also possible to purchase a USB diffuser for your laptop computer. Simply plug the device into the USB port to disperse the essential oil aroma. Consult the manufacturer's guidelines for further information on use.

Personal Inhalers

A personal aromatherapy inhaler is a simple device composed of a case with a glass vial. You add your chosen essential oils to the glass vial and carry the device around with you in your purse or pocket, to inhale as needed. Use a cotton ball (or pad) to absorb the essential oils inside the vial if necessary. There are also variations on this type of inhaler, such as aromasticks (or blank inhalers)—essentially a version of a Vicks inhaler stick.

In addition, you can make your own personal balm using base ingredients of beeswax, cocoa butter, shea butter, vegetable oil base, and essential oils. Add it to a container such as a lip balm tube. Apply to the wrist and temples and inhale as needed. There are various recipes for making aromatherapy balms. The following recipe can be adapted for more complex blends—or consult a certified aromatherapist experienced in making bath and body products for further advice.

Personal Balm Recipe

0.5 oz beeswax
0.25 oz cocoa butter
0.25 oz shea butter
1 oz vegetable oil (for example, sweet almond or jojoba oil)
essential oils (see chart in chapter 11 for amounts)

This recipe makes 10 x 0.15 oz personal balm tubes.

How to Make:

- Heat up water in a small pan on the stove top.
- Add beeswax to a heatproof container.

- Place the container, containing the beeswax, in the water.
- Once the beeswax is melted, add the cocoa butter to the mix.
- Once the cocoa butter is melted, add the shea butter to the mix.
- Once the shea butter is melted, stir together.
- Add in the vegetable oil and stir.
- Take off the heat, add in the essential oils, and stir.
- Quickly pour the liquid into your containers. If you are using lip balm tubes, you will probably want to use a lip balm tray so that you can pour the liquid more efficiently. If the mixture begins to harden before you have finished pouring, reheat it on the stove for a minute.
- Allow the mixture to harden and set.
- Label your tubes with the contents and the date you made them.
- Store in the refrigerator to prolong shelf life, and use within six months.

Baths and Steam Inhalation

It is simple to add a few drops of essential oil directly to warm bath water or disperse in a bath oil. The heat from the water allows for the dispersal of the aroma and is a great way to relax and ease away the stresses of the day. Alternatively, if you are suffering from a head cold or have blocked sinuses or a stuffy nose, fill up a bowl of warm water and add in a few drops of an appropriate essential oil. Cover your head with a towel, lean over the bowl, and inhale the aroma for between five to ten minutes (depending on needs).

Tissues

If you don't have any other type of inhaler or diffuser available, simply add a few drops of essential oil onto a tissue and inhale for a couple of breaths.

Topical

Massage

One of the first ways many people are introduced to the topical application of essential oils is through massage. If you are applying essential oils topically, you need to dilute them in a carrier oil or base before applying them to the skin. In massage, there are various types of carrier oils that are used as a base. Carrier oils for aromatherapy use are vegetable-based oils that have, in general, been cold pressed. Cold-pressed carrier oils retain more of the therapeutic properties of the plant from which they are extracted. Hot-pressed carrier oils contain little, if any, therapeutic properties and are typically used in cooking. Do not use the two types of oils interchangeably.

Popular carrier oils for massage include jojoba, sweet almond, grapeseed, sunflower, and coconut oil, although there are many other types, too. The bulk of a massage oil is made up of carrier oil, with a few drops of essential oils added to it.

Skin Care

Essential oils can also be applied topically through the use of skin-care product bases. These include:

- Oil base
- Lotion base
- Cream base

- Butter base
- Perfume base
- Bath salts base
- Scrub base
- Balm base
- Gel base

Many of the above bases are discussed in chapter 14.

It is *very* important to note that you should always dilute essential oils in a carrier oil or skin-care base before applying them topically to the skin, unless you are a trained professional. Lack of knowledge and experience about an essential oil can lead to the misuse of the oil and may cause skin irritation, sensitization, or allergies, if applied undiluted.

Compresses

You can make a compress with essential oils to assist with pain or inflammation. Fill up a bowl of hot or cold water, add in a few drops of an appropriate essential oil, and soak a small face cloth in the bowl. Squeeze out the excess water and apply the compress to the affected area for several minutes.

14

Essential Oils for Body Care

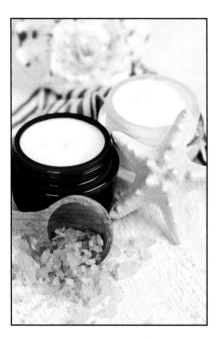

There are a lot of different aromatherapy skin-care products to choose from, and, whether you make your own or buy, you need to understand what actually goes into a therapeutic aromatherapy skin-care product. Many skin-care products claim to contain aromatherapy ingredients, but not all of them contain true essential oils.

Essential oils are the core ingredient of therapeutic aromatherapy products, and your skin type will determine the best type of essential oil blend for you. There are various combinations of essential oils suitable for a particular skin type, but those suggested in this chapter are a great place to start.

Essential oils for body care include the use of essential oils for your body, face, and hair. If you are using essential oils for your face, you will need to remember to decrease the amount of essential oils used because the face is usually more sensitive than other parts of your body. Guidelines on quantities to use, plus tips for blending for essential oils, are given in chapter 11.

Types of Skin and Hair

The skin is the largest organ in the body, and, although some characteristics of your skin type might be determined either by genetics or your age group, others are determined by how you treat your skin. Overexposure to sun and wind, dehydration, and physical injuries all affect the health of your skin. The same is true for your hair, which is also affected by the overuse of hair accessories and styling products. Skin can be divided into different categories. Most people have a combination of both oily and dry skin. For the purpose of this chapter, the recommended essential oils for the different skin types can be used interchangeably with the same categories of hair types.

Dry Skin

Dry skin lacks moisture and is often accompanied by sensitivity. Use essential oils for dry skin with care, particularly if you know that you have sensitive skin, too. It is also advisable to do a "patch" test before using a particular essential oil with which you are unfamiliar. Some essential oils that are suitable for dry skin include:

- Lavender (*Lavandula angustifolia*)
- Patchouli (*Pogostemon cablin*)
- Roman chamomile (*Chamaemelum nobile*)
- Rose (*Rosa damascena*)

Oily Skin

Oily skin is accompanied by problems such as spots and congestion; oily skin is the result of excess sebum production by the sebaceous glands. Teenagers are frequent sufferers. Antiseptic and astringent essential oils are suitable for oily skin and include:

- Geranium (*Pelargonium graveolens*)
- Juniper (*Juniperus communis*)
- Lemon (*Citrus limon*)
- Tea tree (*Melaleuca alternifolia*)

Mature Skin

Mature skin problems often include the development of wrinkles! Essential oils may help reduce wrinkles by stimulating new cell growth through the chemical components that they contain. In addition, combine your chosen essential oils in a carrier oil base that contains a high level of vitamin E. Essential oils for mature skin include:

- Clary sage (*Salvia sclarea*)
- Lavender (*Lavandula angustifolia*)
- Myrrh (*Commiphora myrrha*)
- Neroli (*Citrus aurantium* var. *amara*)
- Rose (*Rosa damascena*)
- Sweet orange (*Citrus aurantium* var. *amara*)

How to Use

The various products recommended as a skin-care base for essential oils are vast. The base for essential oils will depend partially upon personal preference for the consistency and viscosity of a product and partially upon method of application.

Oils

A vegetable-based carrier oil can be used as a bath oil, perfume oil, massage oil, or hot oil treatment for your hair. Choose an appropriate cold-pressed vegetable oil, and add a few drops of essential oil to it. Use in the following ways:

- Bath oil—pour the oil in warm bath water.
- Perfume and massage oil—apply to the skin topically.
- Hot oil treatment for hair—heat up the blended carrier oil and essential oils in a glass container in a microwave oven for fifteen to thirty seconds. Apply to dry hair, cover with a shower cap or towel, and leave on for a minimum of thirty minutes. Remove the shower cap or towel. Add a small amount of shampoo before wetting the hair to enable easier washing. Wash and rinse hair as normal.

Lotions and Creams

Add essential oils to either a white lotion or cream base for regular skin-care use. You can either use a premade, unscented cosmetic base (available from cosmetic suppliers) or make your own from basic ingredients such as beeswax, water, vegetable oil, cocoa butter, and shea butter. Lotions and creams can be used for moisturizing the skin on a daily basis.

The following two recipes are basic recipes for lotions and creams, which can be adapted for more complex blends—or consult a certified aromatherapist experienced in making bath and body products for further advice.

Basic Lotion Recipe

0.6 oz cocoa butter

0.4 oz emulsifying wax

0.8 oz vegetable oil

2.75 oz distilled water

essential oils (see chart in chapter 11 for amounts)

This recipe makes approximately a 5-oz lotion.

How to Make:

- Heat up water in a small pan on the stove top.
- Add cocoa butter to a heatproof container.
- Place the container containing cocoa butter in the water.
- Once the cocoa butter is melted, add the emulsifying wax.
- Once the emulsifying wax is melted, add the vegetable oil.
- Heat up distilled water in a separate small pan on the stove top until warm.
- Take the melted butters/oils and wax off the heat.
- Whisk the mixture, using a hand whisk, on low-medium setting.
- Pour the warm distilled water into the mixture while whisking between five and ten minutes.

- Add the appropriate essential oils.
- Whisk for another ten to twenty seconds.
- Spoon the mixture into an appropriate container.
- Label the container with the contents and the date you made it.
- Store in the refrigerator to prolong shelf life and use within two months.*

Basic Cream Recipe

0.6 oz shea butter
0.6 oz cocoa butter
0.35 oz emulsifying wax
0.1 oz stearic acid
2.65 oz distilled water
essential oils (see chart in chapter 11 for amounts).

This recipe makes approximately a 4-oz cream.

- Heat up water in a small pan on the stove top.
- Add cocoa butter to a heatproof container.
- Place the container containing cocoa butter in the water.
- Once the cocoa butter is melted, add the shea butter.
- Once the shea butter is melted, add the stearic acid and the emulsifying wax.
- Heat up distilled water in a separate small pan on the stove top until warm.
- Take the melted mixture off the heat.
- Whisk the mixture, using a hand whisk, on low-medium setting.

- Pour the warm distilled water into the mixture while whisking between five and ten minutes.
- Add the appropriate essential oils.
- Whisk for a further ten to twenty seconds.
- Spoon the mixture into an appropriate container.
- Label the container with the contents and the date you made it.
- Store in the refrigerator to prolong shelf life and use within two months.*

*As these recipes don't contain any type of preservatives, the shelf life of your product may vary, depending upon how you store it and the introduction of any other potential contaminants into the lotion (for example, unwashed hands).

Butters and Balms

Butters and balms are richer and deeper moisturizing products than lotions and creams. They are a great weekly or monthly treat for the skin. Butters and balms are usually solid at room temperature, although some butters are softer than others. Natural butters, such as shea and cocoa, are extracted from plants but are often combined to make custom aromatherapy butter blends. Balms are made from the combination of various ingredients such as beeswax, vegetable oils, and/or butters. The quantity of each ingredient, and the method used to combine each ingredient, affects the consistency and end result of each product, separating butters and balms from cream and lotion bases.

Scrubs

There are various types of scrubs available for body care, which include:

- Sugar scrub—a scrub that uses sugar as a base. The sugar used is usually brown or white, combined with vegetable oil and essential oils. You can also add in other ingredients like honey and butters. Use as a body scrub.
- Salt scrub—a scrub that uses Epsom, Dead Sea, or sea salt as a base. Combine with vegetable oils and essential oils. Use as a body or foot scrub.
- Combination of sugar and salt scrub.
- Facial scrub—the skin on the face is more sensitive than the rest of the body so use a more gentle scrub base for essential oils, like a combination of ground almonds, ground oatmeal, and essential oils. This type of scrub can also be used as a facial mask. Just add water to combine the ingredients for use.

How to Use a Scrub

- Apply a small amount of the scrub to your wet skin.
- Gently massage in a circular motion, concentrating on any rough areas.
- Leave on for about ten minutes and rinse off the scrub.

CAUTION: Don't use the scrub on your skin if you have sunburn, irritated skin, or cuts.

Bath Salts

Add essential oils to a base of Epsom, Dead Sea, or sea salt; combine and pour a small amount in the bath tub. Bath salts are a great base for allowing the body to soak in warm bath water and can be used to ease aches and pains, too.

Other Bath Products

You can also add essential oils to custom-made bath products, such as bath melts and bath fizzes. These types of bases usually require some knowledge of cosmetic product making, but you can easily learn how to do this by reading a cosmetic product-making book or taking a short course in making your own cosmetic products.

Perfumes

You can add essential oils to perfume sprays, perfume oils, or alcohol-based perfumes, depending upon your preference. Perfume sprays can be used to lightly spritz the face and body, and some like to use these types of sprays to "set" their face makeup. Alcohol-based perfumes, for home use, can be made with a combination base of isopropyl alcohol (90% proof) or an artisan's blend of alcohol, and a small amount of distilled water. However, it can take several weeks for the essential oil perfume to "blend."

Shampoo

Add a couple of drops of essential oils to an unscented shampoo base (available from cosmetic suppliers) for hair care and apply in the usual way.

Gel

Use a base of aloe vera gel for "cooling" down skin that is irritated or has suffered burns. You can also use aloe vera gel as a base for hair gel or add to a hair spray.

15

Essential Oils for Health

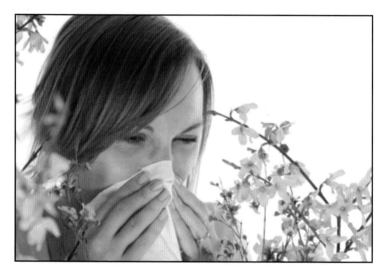

Essential oils can be used to address various health problems. It is always important to understand a person's health history and any medications that they are taking before deciding on a suitable essential oil for a particular problem. In addition, consult your health care practitioner if there are any irregularities in a person's health before using essential oils. Check for contraindications for use, too, as discussed in chapter 11.

The advice in this book is not intended as a substitute for medical advice. However, there are several essential oils that may help with a number of health issues, if you take the time to understand the essential oil first. The suggested essential oils in this chapter are expanded on in *Part Three*.

How to Use

There are various ways in which you can use essential oils for health problems. The most common way is to add the appropriate essential oils to a vegetable oil or lotion base and apply to the body. However, it will depend upon your specific problem, and area of application, as to which method you choose to use. In addition, inhalation by an aromatherapy diffuser, personal inhaler, or a steam inhalation might be more appropriate especially for respiratory difficulties.

Cardiovascular System

The cardiovascular system encompasses both the circulatory and lymphatic systems. Organs and structures such as the heart, arteries, veins, lymph, spleen, and thymus gland are contained within the cardiovascular system. Diseases of the cardiovascular system include heart problems, high/low blood pressure, edema, and glandular fever.

Essential oils for the cardiovascular system include:

- Benzoin (*Styrax benzoin*)
- Black pepper (*Piper nigrum*)
- Cedarwood (*Cedrus atlantica*)
- Roman chamomile (*Chamaemelum nobile*)
- Geranium (*Pelargonium graveolens*)
- Lavender (*Lavandula angustifolia*)
- Neroli (*Citrus aurantium* var. *amara*)
- Rosemary (*Rosmarinus officinalis*)

Digestive System

Organs and structures in the digestive system include the mouth, stomach, intestines, liver, and anus. Diseases of the digestive system include gingivitis, gastritis, ulcers, food poisoning, stomach upsets, flatulence, indigestion, and constipation.

Essential oils for the digestive system include:

- Bergamot (*Citrus bergamia*)
- Cinnamon (*Cinnamomum zeylanicum*)
- Dill (*Anethum graveolens*)
- Fennel (*Foeniculum vulgare*)
- Ginger (*Zingiber officinale*)
- Grapefruit (*Citrus x paradisi*)
- Lemon (*Citrus limon*)
- Sweet orange (*Citrus sinensis*)

Endocrine System

The endocrine system is an extensive network of secretory cells that assist in the correct function of organs and glands in the body, such as the female ovaries. Diseases and imbalances of the endocrine system include menstrual difficulties, menopausal problems, bile production, and thyroid problems.

Essential oils for the endocrine system include:

- Clary sage (*Salvia sclarea*)
- Geranium (*Pelargonium graveolens*)
- Roman chamomile (*Chamaemelum nobile*)
- Clove bud (*Syzygium aromaticum*)
- Cypress (*Cupressus sempervirens*)

- Sweet marjoram (*Origanum majorana*)
- Rose (*Rosa damascena*)
- Rosemary (*Rosmarinus officinalis*)

Immune and Lymphatic System

The immune system is the body's defense system against the invasion of unwanted bacteria and is assisted in this role by various organs of the lymphatic system. Structures and organs in the lymphatic system include lymph, the spleen, and thymus gland. B-lymphocytes and T-lymphocyctes help to provide immunity to the body. Diseases of the lymphatic system include glandular fever; diseases of the immune system include rheumatoid arthritis.

Essential oils for the immune and lymphatic system include:

- Cedarwood (*Cedrus atlantica*)
- Lime (*Citrus aurantifolia*)
- Tea tree (*Melaleuca alternifolia*)
- Myrrh (*Commiphora myrrha*)
- Pine (*Pinus sylvestris*)
- Yarrow (*Achillea millefolium*)

Muscular and Joints System

The muscles and the joints interact with each other to provide freedom of movement within the body. Joints are the site where two or more bones come together. Muscle tissue (skeletal, smooth, and cardiac) provides various functions within the body to allow, for example, facial expression and movement of the back. Diseases and injuries of the muscular and joints system include joint and muscle pain, sprains, lumbago, and rheumatism.

Essential oils for the muscular and joints systems include:

- Roman chamomile (*Chamaemelum nobile*)
- Jasmine (*Jasminum officinale*)
- Juniper (*Juniperus communis*)
- Lavender (*Lavandula angustifolia*)
- Lemon (*Citrus limon*)
- Black pepper (*Piper nigrum*)

Nervous System

The nervous system is the "alert" system that responds to changes both inside and outside the body. It works in conjunction with the endocrine system to bring the body back into balance. Structures and organs within the nervous system include receptors, the brain, spinal cord and nerves, the sympathetic nervous system, and the parasympathetic nervous system. Diseases of the nervous system include stress, depression, dementia, Parkinson's disease, insomnia, migraine, headaches, and neuralgia.

Essential oils for the nervous system include:

- Frankincense (*Boswellia carteri*)
- Melissa (*Melissa officinalis*)
- Neroli (*Citrus aurantium* var. *amara*)
- Patchouli (*Pogostemon cablin*)
- Peppermint (*Mentha piperita*)
- Petitgrain (*Citrus aurantium* var. *amara*)

- Vetiver (*Vetiveria zizanioides*)
- Ylang ylang (*Cananga odorata*)

Reproductive System

The reproductive system covers either the female or male organs of the body, such as the ovaries, uterus, vagina, scrotum, and testes. Diseases of the reproductive system include *Candida albicans*, syphilis, other sexually transmitted diseases, endometritis, and infertility.

Essential oils for the reproductive system include:

- Geranium (*Pelargonium graveolens*)
- Lavender (*Lavandula angustifolia*)
- Rose (*Rosa damascena*)
- Rosemary (*Rosmarinus officinalis*)
- Tea tree (*Melaleuca alternifolia*)
- Myrrh (*Commiphora myrrha*)

Respiratory System

The respiratory system regulates the oxygen that passes through the body and the waste product that it produces for expulsion from the body (carbon dioxide). The chemical reactions derived from the presence of oxygen in the body help the body (and its organs) remain in balance. Various organs and structures play a role in allowing these reactions to take place, including the nose, trachea, lungs, and bronchi. Diseases of the respiratory system include colds, flu, sinusitis, bronchitis, asthma, emphysema, and pneumonia.

Essential oils for the respiratory system include:

- Eucalyptus smithii (*Eucalyptus smithii*)
- Helichrysum (*Helichrysum angustifolium*)
- Lavender (*Lavandula angustifolia*)
- Lemon (*Citrus limon*)
- Myrtle (*Myrtus communis*)
- Thyme (*Thymus vulgaris*)

Urinary System

The urinary system is responsible for the excretion of waste from the body. Organs and structures within the urinary system include the kidneys, the bladder, the ureters, and the urethra. Diseases of the urinary system include kidney stones, bladder infections, cystitis, and incontinence.

Essential oils for the urinary system include:

- Clove (*Syzygium aromaticum*)
- Fennel (*Foeniculum vulgare*)
- Geranium (*Pelargonium graveolens*)
- Rosemary (*Rosmarinus officinalis*)
- Sandalwood (*Santalum album*)
- Tea tree (*Melaleuca alternifolia*)

A Note on Smoking

If you are looking for a bit of natural help to quit smoking, you might consider the use of black pepper (*Piper nigrum*) essential oil. Although there aren't many verifiable clinical research studies on how essential oils may help you to quit smoking, a study carried out by Rose and Behm (1994) indicated that black pepper essential oil helped to decrease cigarette cravings in smokers.

Participants in the study were given cigarette substitutes that delivered either a vapor of black pepper essential oil, a mint/menthol cartridge, or an empty cartridge; those who used the black pepper oil control demonstrated a reduction in cigarette cravings and in symptoms of anxiety and negativity.

If you are trying to quit smoking, try diffusing black pepper via an aromatherapy diffuser, as discussed in chapter 13. You might also want to try diffusing essential oils that help with anxiety symptoms, for example, lavender, neroli, or vetiver. Although these essential oils in themselves will not help you to quit smoking, they might help to ease some of the side effects of cigarette withdrawal. Consult a qualified health-care practitioner for individual advice.

Essential Oils and Health Problems

It is important to view aromatherapy as a complementary rather than an alternative therapy and work in conjunction with the advice of a qualified health professional when choosing the best course of action for a particular problem. Each person presents a different set of circumstances. There are a wide variety of essential oils to choose from for the same problem, and it depends upon a number of variables as to which choice is best for you.

16

Essential Oils for Women

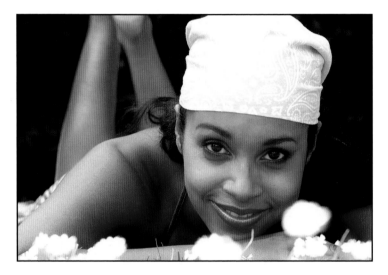

Women deal with a lot of health issues in life that can be aided by the use of essential oils. In addition to skin care, as discussed in chapter 14, there are various stages of a woman's life that can be assisted by essential oils.

Chapter 16 is a brief introduction to the many ways in which a woman can use essential oils from puberty through the later years in life. The suggested essential oils in this chapter are expanded on in *Part Three*.

How to Use

There are various ways in which a woman can use essential oils throughout her life. The most common way is to add the appropriate essential oils to a vegetable oil or lotion base and apply to the body. However, it will depend upon your specific problem and area of application as to which method you choose to use. In addition, inhalation by an aromatherapy diffuser, personal inhaler, or a steam inhalation might be more appropriate, especially for anxiety and stress-related problems.

Essential Oils and Women

Women have a number of essential oils to choose from to help them through the various stages of their lives. If you introduce your daughter, niece, or granddaughter to the use of essential oils in her teenage years, it is likely that she will continue to find benefit from essential oils for the remainder of her life.

Teenage Years

Teenage girls encounter many problems during the transitional journey from child to young woman, and some of these difficulties can affect physical health. In addition, the mental health of a teenage girl can be an emotional roller coaster, causing confusion, depression, and anger. Essential oils may help to control or eliminate some of these difficulties.

Some of the difficulties that teenage girls face, and suggested essential oils for these problems, include:

- The onset of menstruation—frankincense (*Boswellia carteri*), cedarwood (*Cedrus atlantica*), cypress (*Cupressus sempervirens*), Roman chamomile (*Chamaemelum nobile*)
- Acne—petitgrain (*Citrus aurantium* var. *amara*), geranium (*Pelargonium graveolens*)
- Changing body shape (and the lack of confidence or confusion often associated with this)—lemon (*Citrus*

limon), rose (*Rosa damascena*), ylang ylang (*Cananga odorata*)

- Hormonal/mood swings—lavender (*Lavandula angustifolia*), clary sage (*Salvia sclarea*), bergamot (*Citrus bergamia*)
- Exam/study stress—combination of rosemary (*Rosmarinus officinalis*) and lavender (*Lavandula angustifolia*)

Pregnancy

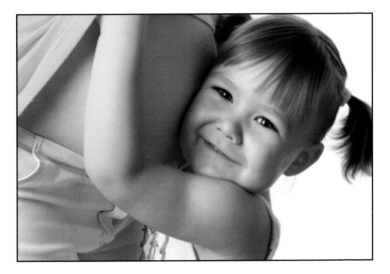

It is *very* important to understand as much as you can about essential oils before using them in pregnancy; where possible, seek professional advice both from a qualified health practitioner and a certified aromatherapist. Although many essential oils can be safely used in pregnancy, there are some essential oils that should never be used (as discussed in chapter 11).

It is usually advisable to avoid all essential oils during the first trimester of pregnancy, particularly if you are at high risk of miscarriage. Although there is no clinical evidence to suggest that essential oils may cause a miscarriage when used in small quantities, some essential oils (for example, hyssop, penny royal) are classed as abortive because of their emmenagogue or abortifacient properties that may stimulate menstruation or premature uterine contractions, respectively. Err on the side of caution if you are unsure of an essential oil reaction.

Essential oils that have a high chemical composition of alcohol are usually more gentle in their actions. Essential oils that are predominately composed of ketones and/or phenols are usually more toxic and should be avoided in pregnancy. Examples include clove (*Syzygium aromaticum*), fennel (*Foeniculum vulgare*), and thyme (*Thymus vulgaris*).

Some of the difficulties faced in pregnancy, and suggested essential oils for these problems, include:

- Morning sickness—petitgrain (*Citrus aurantium* var. *amara*), grapefruit (*Citrus x paradisi*), ginger (*Zingiber officinale*)
- Backache—lavender (*Lavandula angustifolia*), Roman chamomile (*Chamaemelum nobile*)
- Constipation and hemorrhoids—cypress (*Cupressus sempervirens*), frankincense (*Boswellia carteri*), ginger (*Zingiber officinale*)
- Fatigue—bergamot (*Citrus bergamia*), sweet orange (*Citrus sinensis*)
- Stretch marks—lavender (*Lavandula angustifolia*), rose (*Rosa damascena*)

Menopausal Problems

The word "menopause" is a derivation of the Greek words for month, *men*, and halt, *pausis*. Menopause represents the end of one cycle and the start of another in a woman's life. This may last several years and, in some cases, is often preceded by perimenopause.

Menopause is a time when hormonal and physical changes occur in a woman's body and can present a number of problems. These include hot flashes, depression, tiredness, irritability, and changes in skin and hair. If you are taking prescribed medication from a doctor for menopausal problems, or are using hormone replacement therapy (HRT), check with your health practitioner and a certified aromatherapist before using any essential oils in case of any possible interaction.

Some of the difficulties faced in menopause, and suggested essential oils for these problems, include:

- Depression and anxiety—frankincense (*Boswellia carteri*), sweet marjoram (*Origanum marjorana*)
- Insomnia—lavender (*Lavandula angustifolia*), Roman chamomile (*Chamaemelum nobile*), clary sage (*Salvia sclarea*), juniper (*Juniperus communis*)
- Hot flashes and sweating—cypress (*Cupressus sempervirens*), peppermint (*Mentha piperita*), clary sage (*Salvia sclarea*)
- Lack of interest in sex—rose (*Rosa damascena*), ylang ylang (*Cananga odorata*), rosemary (*Rosmarinus officinalis*)

Later Life

Today's "baby boomers" are more active than the previous generation. Life expectancy has increased, too. However, today's aging population still faces a number of difficulties that appear late in life, such as arthritis, rheumatism, poor circulation, and incontinence. For those who suffer, the quality of life can often be improved with the use of essential oils.

If you are taking prescribed medication, check with your health practitioner and a certified aromatherapist before using any essential oils in case of any possible interaction.

Some of the difficulties faced by those in the later years of life, and suggested essential oils for these problems, include:

- Arthritis, rheumatism, and aches and pains—rosemary (*Rosmarinus officinalis*), Roman chamomile (*Chamaemelum nobile*), lavender (*Lavandula angustifolia*), sweet marjoram (*Origanum marjorana*)
- Constipation—ginger (*Zingiber officinale*)
- Diarrhea—peppermint (*Mentha piperita*), lemon (*Citrus limon*)
- Incontinence—cypress (*Cupressus sempervirens*).
- Poor circulation—clary sage (*Salvia sclarea*), lemon (*Citrus limon*)
- Influenza—eucalyptus (*Eucalyptus smithii*), lemon (*Citrus limon*)
- Dementia* and forgetfulness—rosemary (*Rosmarinus officinalis*), peppermint (*Mentha piperita*)

*Note, essential oils cannot cure diseases such as dementia but may help cope with some of the effects.

17

Essential Oils for Babies and Children

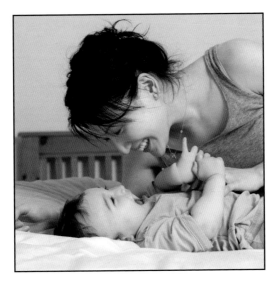

Babies and young children are usually receptive to new ideas, and introducing essential oils at such a young age will open up a new world. However, it is important to understand that not only are some essential oils not advised for use with this age group, but less is always more when it comes to quantity. Follow these guidelines along with the professional advice of a certified aromatherapist who has training in the area, and you should be able to use essential oils both safely and happily with baby and child.

How to Use

There are various ways in which you can use essential oils with babies. If your child is under two years of age, choose an unscented white lotion base over a carrier oil, as it is more easily absorbed by baby's young skin. In addition, an oily baby can wriggle free more easily! Never apply an essential oil to a baby's skin without diluting it first.

The amount of essential oil to use in the lotion base depends, in part, upon the essential oil. However, safe use for a baby is usually up to two drops of essential oil per ounce of carrier lotion. Consult a certified aromatherapist for more specific advice on a particular problem, including any contraindicators for use.

In addition to using lotions for massage, you can use one to two drops of essential oil diluted in water and spray around the baby's sleeping area before going to sleep. Lavender sachets are also a good idea to slip inside a pillowcase or place by the baby's crib. You can also add a drop of essential oil to an unscented bath lotion or bubble base for general skin-care at bath time. Use an aromatherapy diffuser in your baby's or child's room for sleep or cold difficulties.

Finally, never use essential oils internally with a baby or young child, and keep them away from their eyes. As an alternative to essential oils, use hydrosols, which are more gentle in nature.

Babies, Aroma, and Massage

Babies identify the world around them using smell. Studies have shown that smells "inhaled" by a baby, via the amniotic fluid in the prenatal stage, are the smells preferred after birth, too (Davis and Porter 1991). If mom uses certain essential oils in her pregnancy, the baby should learn to recognize those smells on arrival into the world.

Massage for babies was a traditional skill that was passed down from grandmother to mother, a skill that has more or less been forgotten in today's modern world. Some new mothers are encouraged to rediscover this skill by forward-thinking health professionals, but massage is still perceived more as a luxury than a necessity for health. Massage helps to affirm a strong bond between mom and child. Add essential oils to the equation, and the whole experience becomes beneficial for both, helping to ensure a good night's sleep, in addition to the skin-care benefits for the baby.

There are various other ways in which aroma can benefit babies, for example, the use of sachets and sprays. You can use aromatherapy with babies for such problems as teething, crying, colds, clinginess, eczema, and anxiety.

Safe Essential Oils for Baby
Although you need to understand both the problem and the essential oil before choosing an essential oil for a baby, the following essential oils are generally considered gentle enough for use:

- Bergamot (*Citrus bergamia*)
- Roman chamomile (*Chamaemelum nobile*)
- Eucalyptus smithii (*Eucalyptus smithii*)
- Frankincense (*Boswellia carteri*)
- Geranium (*Pelargonium graveolens*)
- Ginger (*Zingiber officinale*)
- Grapefruit (*Citrus x paradisi*)
- Lavender (*Lavandula angustifolia*)
- Lemon (*Citrus limon*)

- Mandarin (*Citrus reticulata*)
- Rose (*Rosa damascena*)
- Sweet orange (*Citrus sinensis*)
- Tea tree (*Melaleuca alternifolia*)

Essential Oils to Avoid

The following essential oils should always be avoided with a baby for one reason or another. This is only intended as a general guideline, and you should check with a certified aromatherapist for further information:

- Peppermint (*Mentha piperita*) and cornmint (*Mentha arvensis*)—high in menthone, which is too much for a baby's respiratory system to cope with, up to and including the age of three years.
- Hyssop (*Hyssop officinalis*)—use only under professional guidance due to chemical components.
- Basil (*Ocimum basilicum*)—do not use the chemotype which is high in phenols; choose the linalool chemotype.
- Juniper (*Juniperus communis*)—use only under professional guidance for children and never with babies.

Essential Oils for Specific Problems

Each baby and child is different, and if you are concerned about a specific problem, it is advisable to consult a certified aromatherapist with specific training. However, the following essential oils are suggested for the problems outlined below:

- Baby skin care—rose (*Rosa damascena*)
- Chicken pox—Roman chamomile (*Chamaemelum nobile*), lavender (*Lavandula angustifolia*), peppermint (*Mentha piperita*)*

- Chest infections—sweet marjoram (*Origanum marjorana*)
- Confidence booster for young children who are clingy—lemon (*Citrus limon*)
- Digestive problems—sweet orange (*Citrus sinensis*)
- Eczema—geranium (*Pelargonium graveolens*), lavender (*Lavandula angustifolia*), bergamot (*Citrus bergamia*)
- Teething problems—Roman chamomile (*Chamaemelum nobile*)

*Use only with a child over three years of age and under the guidance of a certified aromatherapist.

18

Essential Oils for the Home

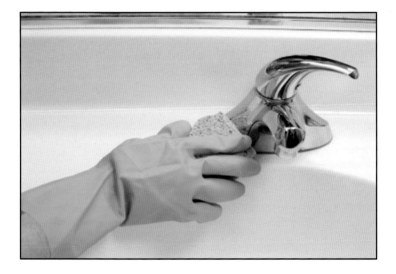

Essential oils can be used to protect both your home and yourself in your home. Many essential oils have bactericidal properties and can replace manufactured cleaning products in the house-cleaning process. In addition, it is also useful to have a ready-to-go first-aid kit of essential oils in case of emergency, such as a burn or a bee sting.

Lavender (*Lavandula angustifolia*) is probably the most valuable essential oil to have in your home for a number of reasons. It is versatile in its use, it is gentle to use with babies and young children, and it is one of the few essential oils that can be used undiluted (when directed to do so by a suitably qualified professional).

Bactericidal Essential Oils

Most essential oils contain bactericidal properties, albeit some deal with different types of bacteria more efficiently than others. Many contain antiseptic, antiviral, and antifungal properties, too, all of which are useful to combat the growth of bacteria and dirt within your home. In addition, essential oils that are approaching their "sell-by" date, with regard to skin care, can be used as cleaning agents. The essential oils discussed in this chapter are all assumed to have antibacterial properties, with additional, relevant properties listed where appropriate.

Air Fresheners

You can purify the air within your home with the use of an aromatherapy diffuser or make up a simple spray. Certain essential oils will leave your home smelling both fresh and clean, in addition to purifying the air of unwanted bacteria.

Herbs such as rosemary (*Rosmarinus officinalis*), clove (*Syzygium aromaticum*), and thyme (*Thymus vulgaris*) were used to protect people against the Black Death in medieval times. Doctors in particular wore masks (shaped like a beak) that contained herbs that they believed would protect them from contracting the disease from their patients. In addition, it was once common practice to cleanse the air in hospitals and sick rooms with the burning of appropriate herbs to prevent the spread of infection.

Suitable essential oils for cleansing the air in your home include:

- Eucalyptus (*Eucalyptus smithii*)—antiseptic, antiviral
- Fennel (*Foeniculum vulgare*)—antiseptic, antimicrobial
- Rosemary (*Rosmarinus officinalis*)—antiseptic, antimicrobial, antifungal.

Add approximately fifteen drops of essential oil to one ounce of water to use the essential oil in a spray. Consult the instructions on your aromatherapy diffuser for quantities of essential oil to use.

Cleaning Your Home

You can use essential oils to clean all aspects of your home, including the following:

- Lavender (*Lavandula angustifolia*)—antimicrobial, antiseptic
- Lemon (*Citrus limon*)—antiseptic, antimicrobial
- Lime (*Citrus aurantifolia*)—antiseptic, antiviral, anti bacterial
- Pine (*Pinus sylvestris*)—antimicrobial, antiseptic, antiviral
- Thyme (*Thymus vulgaris*)—antimicrobial, antiseptic, antifungal

Although all of these essential oils can be used to both wipe down kitchen and bathroom work spaces, and the bedroom and living areas, you might prefer to use an essential oil such as lavender in the bedroom and an essential oil such as pine in the kitchen.

You can also use these essential oils for wiping down chopping boards: add a drop or two of essential oil to your dishcloth or sponge, and wipe down the board. To use essential oils to wipe down work tops, add your chosen blend of essential oils to a pail or bowl of warm water, depending on the size of the surface area you are cleaning. In general, you can add up to fifteen drops of essential oil to an average-sized pail.

Caring for Your Floor

If you want to make a natural carpet freshener, add one drop of essential oil to one tablespoon of bicarbonate of soda and sprinkle on the carpet before vacuuming. Essential oils are also handy to have around if you have a pet who is prone to having unwanted "accidents" in the house. Wipe down the affected area in the same way as recommended for wiping down kitchen and bathroom work surfaces. However, if you have a carpet or flooring cover that requires particular care, consult a specialist first.

Laundry Tip

Add a few drops of tea tree (*Melaleuca alternifolia*) or eucalyptus (*Eucalyptus smithii*) essential oil to your bed linen in the washing machine before switching it on. Not only will your bed linen smell fresh and clean, the antibacterial properties of the essential oils will help to protect against bacteria.

First-Aid Kit for Your Home

A first-aid kit of ready-to-go essential oils is a great tool to have around the home in case of minor accidents. A basic first-aid kit of essential oils includes:

- Clove (*Syzygium aromaticum*)—for cuts, burns, insect repellent, toothache, colds, flu
- Geranium (*Pelargonium graveolens*)—for burns, bruises, stress
- Ginger (*Zingiber officinale*)—for diarrhea, indigestion, nausea, fatigue, pain
- Lavender (*Lavandula angustifolia*)—for cuts, burns, insect bites and stings, sunburn
- Lemon (*Citrus limon*) or lime (*Citrus aurantifolia*)—for chilblains, corns, dyspepsia, colds, flu, fever
- Peppermint (*Mentha piperita*)—for toothache, muscle pain, flatulence, nausea, migraine, stress, fatigue
- Roman chamomile (*Chamaemelum nobile*)—for cuts, earache, insect bites, teething pain (babies), toothache, inflammation, insomnia, headache
- Tea tree (*Melaleuca alternifolia*)—for burns, cold sores, wounds, chicken pox, colds, flu

Additional base products to have in your first-aid kit include:

- Distilled water
- Unscented white lotion base
- Basic vegetable oil
- Hydrosol
- Aloe vera gel
- Empty, and clean, bottles and jars to make up an appropriate blend as needed

Store your first-aid kit in a safe, cool, dark place in order to have it ready when you need it. Check the contents once in a while to ensure products are not out of date or in need of replacing.

Essential Oils for Shock, Accidents, and Bereavement

Sometimes, there is a sudden shock, accident, or bereavement in your life that knocks you off your feet. Upon hearing such news, it is useful to have one of the following essential oils available, as an addition to your basic first-aid kit of essential oils, as they are known for their calming properties and their ability to help in stressful situations:

- Neroli (*Citrus aurantium* var. *amara*)
- Peppermint (*Mentha piperita*)
- Vetiver (*Vetiveria zizaniodes*)

Use the chosen essential oil via one of the inhalation methods, as discussed in chapter 13.

19

Essential Oils for Travel

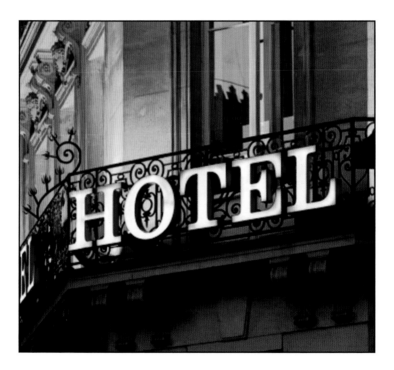

Vacation time often means traveling away from home to unfamiliar places. Although fun, travel can sometimes incur some unexpected problems, including travel sickness, sunburn, stomach upsets, and insect bites. Minor problems can be addressed with a well-planned essential oil kit, put together before you leave home. For more serious issues, consult a health professional.

Motion Sickness

Motion sickness can occur whether you're traveling by train, plane, boat, or car, and at any age, too. Two essential oils you should have in your essential oil travel kit are peppermint (*Mentha piperita*) and ginger (*Zingiber officinale*). Both have therapeutic properties to help relieve the feeling of nausea and sickness.

One of the most effective methods for using essential oils for motion sickness is inhalation. Add a drop of essential oil to a tissue and inhale, or use a personal inhaler. Alternatively, if you are traveling by car, add a drop of essential oil to a plug-in car diffuser. You can also blend the essential oil with a carrier oil or lotion base prior to your journey, and massage the stomach and upper abdomen as needed.

Jet Lag

Depending upon how far you are traveling, and how many time zones you are crossing on your flight, it might take a few days for your body to get back into its natural rhythm both on arrival at your destination and on the return trip home. Flying east is supposed to be more difficult in terms of adjustment than flying westwards. The circadian rhythm of your body becomes unbalanced during long-haul flights, and consequently your digestive and sleep patterns become out of synchronization. The same is similar for night-shift workers.

Use grapefruit (*Citrus x paradisi*) essential oil on arrival to help keep your mind focused and alert while adjusting to the different time zone. You can also combine grapefruit essential oil with lavender (*Lavandula angustifolia*) essential oil in bath salts for a relaxing bath. Another great essential oil to use is geranium (*Pelargonium graveolens*).

Minor Stomach Upsets

Minor stomach upsets often occur on vacation due to a change in diet or the type of water. Both peppermint and ginger essential oils may help to relieve the symptoms of minor stomach upsets. In addition, use lemon (*Citrus limon*) essential oil for acidic disorders. Prepare a carrier lotion or oil with the appropriate essential oils before traveling. Massage over the abdomen as required.

Sunburn

Sunburn causes soreness, redness, and inflammation. It is sensible to protect yourself against the intense heat and sun, but, if you still get caught out, try lavender, Roman chamomile, peppermint, or geranium essential oils. Combine the appropriate oils in a white lotion base, which is more soothing than a carrier oil, and apply to the affected areas with care.

Insect Bites

Insects, such as mosquitoes, can cause nasty and painful bites, if left untreated. Apply citronella (*Cymbopogon nardus*) or lemongrass (*Cymbopogon citratus*) essential oils to the skin in a carrier oil base, or in a spray, before going outside. Use lavender, tea tree, eucalyptus, or geranium essential oils to relieve the itching and pain caused by insect bites. Combine one or more of these essential oils in a white lotion base, and apply to the affected area.

Traveling with Essential Oils on Planes

Travel and flight restrictions vary from country to country, but, within the United States, the 3-1-1 rule for carry-ons applies. Simply put, you can carry a limited amount of liquids on board the aircraft with you. This means that you have to check in your essential oils and essential oil blends as checked luggage, or make sure you are within the 3-1-1 rule. Current regulations specify that you can carry liquids on board the aircraft provided that liquids are contained in a 3.4-ounce bottle or smaller, and all bottles have to fit inside a single one-quart bag (per traveler). The bag has to be available for separate x-ray by security personnel.

Making Up an Essential Oil Kit for Travel

You can make up an essential oil kit of essential oils and blends before you travel, depending upon where you travel, for how long, and what your particular problems are. Your pre-prepared kit may vary, but I find that the following mix of essential oils and blends works well. In addition, this size of kit meets the current requirements of the 3-1-1 rule for carry-ons:

- Motion sickness—personal inhaler of either peppermint or ginger essential oil
- Jet lag—one ounce white lotion blend of grapefruit and geranium essential oils
- Minor stomach upsets—one ounce white lotion blend of peppermint, ginger, or lemon essential oils
- Sunburn and insect bites—one ounce white lotion blend of lavender essential oil
- Insect spray—one ounce spray of citronella essential oil
- General—0.5 ounce bottle of any type of additional, and appropriate, essential oil for the inhaler as necessary

Suggested bases for using essential oils for travel include a simple white lotion base or aloe vera gel. Aloe vera gel is especially useful and soothing for burns and after-sun treatments.

Safe Travel with Essential Oils

If you plan ahead in making your aromatherapy travel kit, you should have all the necessary essential oils and blends for any minor emergency that might occur when traveling. Just remember to check current security restrictions and store your essential oils appropriately. Keep them away from intense heat and light at your destination.

20

Social, Seasonal, and Practical Uses

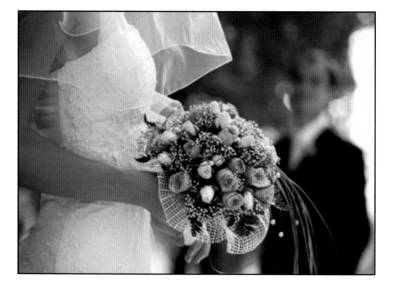

Essential oils can be used for many different occasions in your life, both at work and at play. Essential oils for work and study can help you to get the job done more efficiently and quickly, whereas essential oils for social occasions, such as weddings, parties, and other celebrations, can help to set the mood and encourage your guests to socialize. In addition, you can add in a seasonal element. For example, celebrate Christmas and the holidays with spicy, base note essential oils, or celebrate summer with citrus, top note essential oils.

You can also use some essential oils to help alleviate your pet's problems. Although verifiable research in this area is almost non-existent, some aromatherapists have successfully used aroma-therapy with pets. However, I advise both caution and common sense when using essential oils with pets, as animals react differently to essential oils than humans do.

Essential Oils for All Occasions

Essential oils can be used in many areas of your life, outside of home and health care. This chapter contains some fun and inventive ideas, based on experience and practice. In addition, this chapter gives you an excellent starting point to make your life, both at work and play, successful and fun and to help your pets enjoy a more healthy life, too!

Essential Oils at Work

Work can take its toll on your health, both physically and mentally. In addition to the stress of meeting deadlines, environmental factors can influence how you feel, too. It is not always possible to request an improvement in your working conditions, so the use of appropriate essential oils may help improve the situation temporarily. However, if you work with other people within an office or retail space, always ask before diffusing essential oils in the air, as you might not be aware of special medical considerations of others.

Essential oils suitable for diffusing in the office to lift mood include:

- Citrus essential oils—lemon (*Citrus limon*), lime (*Citrus aurantifolia*), grapefruit (*Citrus x paradisi*), sweet orange (*Citrus sinensis*), bergamot (*Citrus bergamia*)
- Rosemary (*Rosmarinus officinalis*)

A 2003 study on rosemary and lavender essential oils showed that rosemary essential oil increased both work performance and quality of memory (Moss et al. 2003). A 2008 study on lemon and lavender essential oils demonstrated that lemon oil enhanced positive mood, and norepinephrine levels were elevated (Kiecolt-Glaser et al. 2008).

The most effective way to use these essential oils at work is with the diffusion or inhalation methods discussed in chapter 13.

Essential Oils for Students

According to the great William Shakespeare (1564–1616), "There's rosemary, that's for remembrance" (*Hamlet*, Act IV, Scene Five). Students today, whether they study Shakespeare or not, may benefit from taking this piece of advice: rosemary (*Rosamarinus officinalis*) is one of the most recommended essential oils as an aid to increase memory. In addition, peppermint (*Mentha piperita*) is suggested for mental fatigue (Moss et al. 2008). Spanish sage (*Salvia lavandulifolia*) is recommended as an aid to improve both mood and memory (Tildesley et al. 2005). Essential oils suggested for students for studying and exams can also be used as an aid for job interviews.

Essential Oils for Yoga

Yoga is an increasingly popular practice in today's fast-paced world, and, although yoga in itself can help relieve the symptoms of stress, you can combine your yoga practice with the diffusion of appropriate essential oils. Part of yoga practice is the ability to meditate and ground the body. Appropriate grounding essential oils that may help with meditation include:

- Cedarwood (*Cedrus atlantica*)
- Frankincense (*Boswellia carteri*)
- Patchouli (*Pogostemon cablin*)
- Vetiver (*Vetiveria zizanioides*)
- Sandalwood (*Santalum album*)

In addition to diffusing essential oils during your yoga practice, you can wipe down your yoga mat, at the end of your practice, with a blend of antibacterial essential oils. Combine appropriate essential oils in a spray bottle with water, and mist down your mat. Use tea tree (*Melaleuca alternifolia*), lemon (*Citrus limon*), and thyme (*Thymus vulgaris*).

Essential Oils for Weddings

Flowers have enjoyed a long association with love and have been used in weddings for centuries. Lavender (*Lavandula angustifolia*) and sweet marjoram (*Origanum marjorana*) have both been used as an ingredient in love potions. Rosemary (*Rosmarinus officinalis*) was once entwined in the bridal crown of Greek brides. In England, flower girls are traditional at weddings; an age-old tradition dictates that a flower girl precedes the bride down the pathway to the church, scattering flower blossoms as she goes, in order that the bride enjoys a lifetime of happiness and flowers.

It is now possible to custom scent your wedding in a way similar to which brides color coordinate their wedding. Essential oils are versatile in their wedding use, and, although it often comes down to personal preference for a particular scent, essential oils with aphrodisiac properties are the most suitable choice for weddings! Aphrodisiac essential oils include:

- Neroli (*Citrus aurantium* var. *amara*)
- Patchouli (*Pogostemon cablin*)
- Rose (*Rosa damascena*)
- Sandalwood (*Santalum album*)
- Ylang ylang (*Cananga odorata*)

You can choose to use your essential oil scent in a candle, massage oil, lotion, or spritzer base. Make a custom scent "theme" throughout your wedding, for example, as a bride's personal fragrance on her wedding day, for candles at the wedding reception, and as favors for your wedding guests. An aromatherapist who has experience in this area will be able to advise you of suitable choices for your wedding day.

Essential Oils for Parties and Celebrations

You can enhance your parties and celebrations with the use of essential oils in candles and diffusers. Your choice of essential oils will depend on the aim of your party or gathering. Do you want to set the scene for love, get more social, or chill out? The following essential oils are listed with the suggested use for your party or celebration, taking into account the therapeutic properties of each essential oil:

- Romantic mood—rose (*Rosa damascena*), ylang ylang (*Cananga odorata*), neroli (*Citrus aurantium* var. *amara*), sandalwood (*Santalum album*)
- Conversation starters/social mingling—peppermint (*Mentha piperita*), grapefruit (*Citrus x paradisi*), sweet orange (*Citrus aurantium*), lemon (*Citrus limon*)

- Relaxing mood—myrrh (*Commiphora myrrha*), frankincense (*Boswellia carteri*), lavender (*Lavandula angustifolia*), geranium (*Pelargonium graveolens*)

Essential Oils for Seasons

Certain seasons often dictate a preference for one essential oil over another, depending on the circumstances, your health, and your mood. As winter approaches, the thought of warming, spice oils seems more comforting than light citrus essential oils, which are appealing in summer. However, often the two can be combined, like cinnamon (*Cinnamomum zeylanicum*) and sweet orange (*Citrus sinensis*).

The most useful way for using essential oils seasonally is through an aromatherapy diffuser, which can help to set a particular mood for your home. You can also adapt each blend for personal use in lotions, sprays, and oils, depending upon your preference.

Essential Oils for Pets

My experience using essential oils with pets is limited to use with my own dog. Dogs, in addition to horses, probably obtain the most benefit from the use of essential oils. Use with cats is limited because of the potential for toxicity. Other animals may benefit from essential oils, too, but it is best to check with a certified aromatherapist who has experience with working with such animals—and a veterinarian who understands essential oils.

Using essential oils with pets can be beneficial, depending both on the animal species and the animal's receptiveness to the oil. According to Kristen Leigh Bell in *Holistic Aromatherapy for*

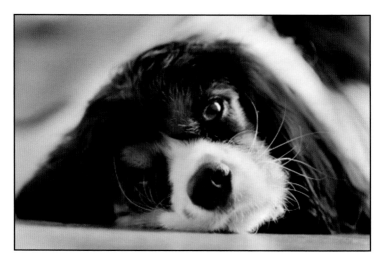

Animals, essential oils act on a physical, emotional, spiritual, and conditional level with animals—although the physical level is the most important factor.

How to Introduce Your Pet to Essential Oils

Pets are, in some respects, like children. They might be more open to one aroma than another. Try a "sniff test" with your pet first to see how he reacts to it. Pets have different personalities, too—so just because one pet reacts in a positive way to a scent, doesn't mean that another pet will do likewise.

An animal's physiological makeup is also different from a human's, something to bear in mind when considering how an animal might react to an essential oil on a physical level.

Essential Oils for Dogs

My dog *loves* the aroma of essential oils! He has no difficulty in "sniff testing" all of the aromas around him! He has been exposed to the scent of many essential oils in our home since he was four months old, so his receptiveness to them has probably increased, to some extent, more so than the average dog. However, a dog's sense of smell is much greater than a human's, and, therefore, aromatherapy might just be the right type of therapy to try with your dog.

I have successfully used essential oils to help my dog with these conditions. The amounts quoted are based on my personal experience and the size of my dog (who weighs approximately twenty-five pounds):

- Ant bites – use a warm compress with lavender (*Lavandula angustifolia*) essential oil and hold over the affected area for a few minutes. Add one to two drops of essential oil to a face-cloth–sized compress. Repeat and increase if necessary.
- Cracked paw pads – apply a small amount of white lotion to the area with an essential oil like lavender (*Lavandula angustofolia*). Use one to two drops of essential oil to half an ounce of lotion. Wrap the paw in a towel for five minutes to allow the lotion to soak in and to avoid your dog from licking off the lotion.
- Bed freshener – use an essential oil spray to freshen up your dog's sleeping area. Use up to five drops per ounce of water. A lavender hydrosol is also a great alternative.
- Disinfectant – essential oils are safe to use in your home with pets, if you follow the guidelines for doing so. If your dog is sick, use a disinfectant blend of essential oils to clean down the area, as discussed in chapter 18.
- Shampoo – a dog's skin pH level is different from that of a human, so it is important to use the right type of

essential oil shampoo when bathing your dog. Purchase a preblended mix of essential oil shampoo that has been formulated for dogs. The important thing to remember is not to substitute your own shampoo for your dog's shampoo.

- Anxiety – many dogs suffer from anxiety, for example, separation anxiety, anxiety brought on by a visit to the veterinarian's office, or thunderstorms. Diffuse a calming blend of essential oils in your home or area where the dog is contained, or gently mist the air around him with a spray.

Hydrosols are also a good alternative to using essential oils.

Essential Oils for Cats

Cats are very different from dogs, in more ways than one. A cat's physiological makeup is different from that of a dog, most notably in how a cat's liver works. A cat's liver does not break down substances in the same way, and therefore there is the potential to build up more toxicity in the system. Bell writes in her book that cats are more sensitive—and have the potential for greater toxicity—when exposed to certain chemical components in essential oils. For example, chemical components present in citrus and pine essential oils—limonene and pinene—may cause a greater adverse reaction in cats.

Although there is limited research on potential toxicity in using essential oils with cats, extreme caution is usually advised. Again, a hydrosol might be a safer alternative for using with cats, although there is little recorded evidence to prove or disprove the safe use of either product.

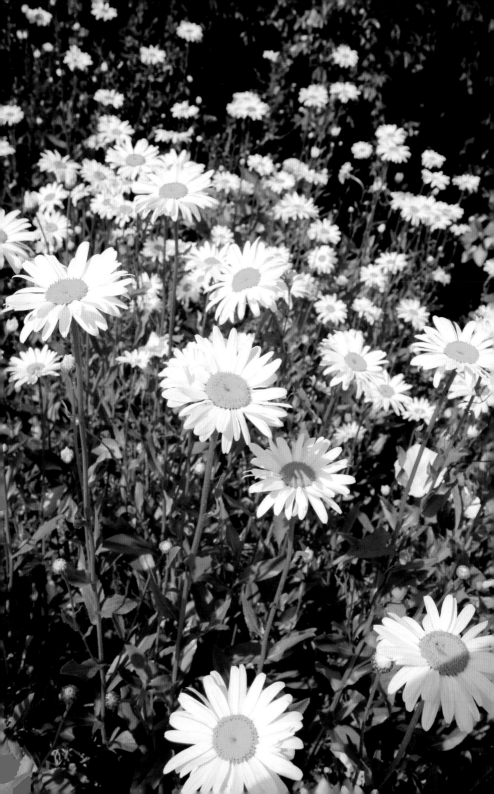

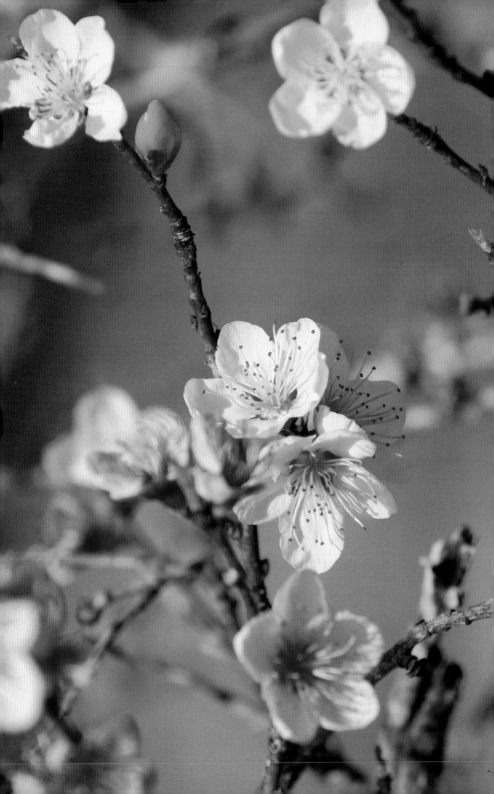

Part Three

Essential Oils Reference Guide

How to Use the Essential Oils Reference Guide

The *Essential Oils Reference Guide* part of this book is intended as a general reference guide to those essential oils highlighted throughout the book. In addition to using this guide, refer to other sections of the book and specific professional advice pertaining to your situation before using any of the essential oils listed.

Uses for each grouping or task are suggested where appropriate. It was not always possible to make specific suggestions for the use of each essential oil as some essential oils lend themselves to specific groupings or tasks better than others.

Alternative Essential Oils

Each essential oil profile has suggestions for alternative essential oils. Alternative essential oils are suggested on the basis of:

- Similar chemical makeup of the essential oil
- Aroma of the essential oil
- Main therapeutic properties

However, alternative essential oils are not exact replicas of the original essential oil profiled. Sometimes, it was not possible to match all of the above factors to each essential oil. In these cases, I used my personal experience and training to arrive at some of the suggestions.

Cost

The final point in each essential oil profile lists cost, represented by the US dollar sign. Again, this is intended as a guideline only, as individual costs vary between suppliers, seasons, chemotypes, and other factors. However, it does represent a fair starting point for what to expect with regard to the pricing of a true essential oil. The costing of each essential oil is determined as follows:

- $ = under $20
- $$ = between $20 and $50
- $$$ = over $50

The costing is based on 1/3 ounce (10 ml) and is an approximate guide only.

Benzoin

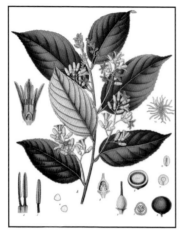

Botanical Name: *Styrax benzoin.*
Synonyms: Gum benzoin.
Botanical Family: *Styracaceae.*
Note: Base.
Blends Well with: Base note spice and floral oils, in addition to top note citrus oils; also peppermint.
Alternative Oils: Jasmine (*Jasminum officinale*), vanilla (*Vanilla planifolia*).
Method of Extraction: A crude resin (not essential oil) is collected from the tree. The crude resin materializes as brittle lumps, exuded from the tree when it is cut. The appearance of the resin is gray-brown with red streaks. It is collected and used to make a resinoid or resin absolute.

Distribution of Plant: A tree that is native to Indonesia. Sumatra benzoin is native specifically to Sumatra.

Description of Plant: A large, tropical tree, which grows up to sixty-five feet in height. It has white, pendulous flowers, citrus-like leaves, and a hard shell fruit.

Characteristics of Essential Oil: Orange-brown in color with a sweet balsamic aroma resembling vanilla, with slight chocolate undertones. It is thick and viscous in nature.

Main Chemical Components of Essential Oil: Esters.

Main Therapeutic Properties of Essential Oil: Anti-inflammatory, antiseptic, astringent, expectorant, sedative.

Uses for Body Care: Inflamed and irritated skin, dry and cracked skin.

Uses for Health: Arthritis, asthma, bronchitis, stress, depression.

Uses for Women: Cystitis.

Uses for Babies and Children: Sun cream (after care).

Use for the Home: Air freshener.

Use for Travel: Sunburn.

Social and Seasonal Use: Parties, celebrations, winter blends.

Ways to Use: Massage oils, diffusers, skin-care bases (scrubs, lotions, creams, butters, balms), perfume base, sprays, bath products (oils, fizzes, melts, salts), candles.

Cautions: No known contraindications for general aromatherapy use. Do not confuse with Siam benzoin, which is also used in perfumery. Sumatra benzoin is native to Sumatra (and Malaysia), whereas Siam benzoin is native to Thailand, Cambodia, and Vietnam.

Cost: $

Bergamot

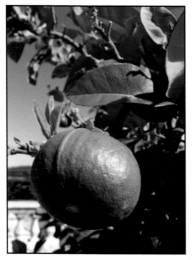

Botanical Name: *Citrus bergamia.*

Synonyms: *Citrus aurantium* subsp. *Bergamia.*

Botanical Family: *Rutaceae.*

Note: Top.

Blends Well with: Other citrus essential oils, jasmine, peppermint, lavender, base note tree essential oils, geranium, eucalyptus.

Alternative Oils: Petitgrain (*Citrus aurantium* var. *amara*), mandarin (*Citrus reticulata*), sweet orange (*Citrus sinensis*).

Method of Extraction: Cold expression of the fruit peel.

Distribution of Plant: Native to tropical Asia, but today it is predominately grown in Calabria, Italy.

Description of Plant: An average-sized tree that grows up to fifteen feet in height. The fruit resembles an orange in appearance, but the color of bergamot fruit ripens from green to yellow.

Characteristics of Essential Oil: Pale green-yellow in color. It has a fresh, citrus aroma.

Main Chemical Components of Essential Oil: Esters, monoterpenes, and alcohols.

Main Therapeutic Properties of Essential Oil: Analgesic, antiseptic, antidepressant, antiviral, digestive, diuretic.

Uses for Body Care: Oily skin, inflamed skin, psoriasis, acne, eczema.

Uses for Health: Indigestion, flatulence, colds, flu, anxiety, depression.

Uses for Women: Severe mood swings, lack of confidence.

Uses for Babies and Children: Uplifting and gentle.

Use for the Home: Air freshener, shock.

Use for Travel: Insect repellent.

Social and Seasonal Use: Parties, celebrations, spring blends.

Ways to Use: Massage oils, diffusers, skin-care bases (scrubs, lotions, creams, butters, balms), sprays, candles.

Cautions: Phototoxic. Use with care prior to exposure to the sun or ultraviolet light to avoid severe burning and skin sensitivities.

Cost: $

Cedarwood

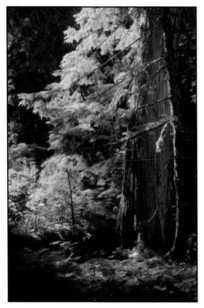

Botanical Name: *Cedrus atlantica.*

Synonyms: Atlantic cedar, Moroccan cedarwood, Atlas cedar, cedar.

Botanical Family: *Pinaceae.*

Note: Base.

Blends Well with: Other base note tree essential oils, bergamot, neroli, vetiver, some citrus note essential oils, lavender.

Alternative Oils: Texas cedar (*Juniperus ashei*), myrrh (*Commiphora myrrha*).

Method of Extraction: Steam distillation of the wood.

Distribution of Plant: Native to the Atlas mountains of Algeria and Morocco.

Description of Plant: A tall, evergreen tree that grows up to 130 feet in height. It is shaped like a pyramid. The wood is highly aromatic.

Characteristics of Essential Oil: Yellow or amber in color. It has a warm, woody, camphoraceous aroma.

Main Chemical Components of Essential Oil: Sesquiterpenes, alcohols, and ketones.

Main Therapeutic Properties of Essential Oil: Antiseptic, aphrodisiac, astringent, antibacterial, expectorant, and sedative.

Uses for Body Care: Oily skin, dry skin, eczema, dermatitis, adult and teenage acne.

Uses for Health: Arthritis, bronchitis, stress, coughs.

Uses for Babies and Children: Eczema, inflammation.

Use for the Home: Air freshener.

Use for Travel: Skin care.

Social and Seasonal Use: Yoga, weddings, parties, celebrations, winter blends.

Ways to Use: Massage oils, diffusers, skin-care bases (scrubs, lotions, creams, butters, balms), perfume base, sprays, bath products (oils, fizzes, melts, salts), candles. Also available as a hydrosol (depending upon specific species).

Cautions: Avoid in pregnancy.

Cost: $

Chamomile (Roman)

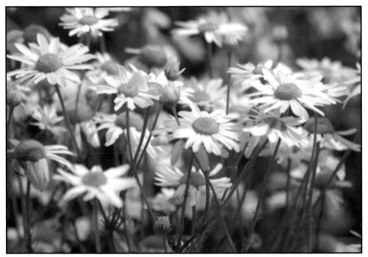

Botanical Name: *Chamaemelum nobile.*

Synonyms: *Anthemis noblis,* true chamomile, English chamomile, chamomile, camomile.

Botanical Family: *Asteraceae.*

Note: Middle.

Blends Well with: Lavender, neroli, cypress.

Alternative Oils: German chamomile (*Matricaria recutica*).

Method of Extraction: Steam distillation of the flowers.

Distribution of Plant: Native to southern Europe. Roman chamomile is now also cultivated in the United States, the United Kingdom, France, and Italy.

Description of Plant: A small, perennial herb that very much resembles a daisy in appearance with its white, daisy-like flowers. It also has feathery leaves.

Characteristics of Essential Oil: Pale yellow in color (with a tinge of blue). It turns more yellow, the longer you keep it. Its botanical cousin, German chamomile (*Matricaria recutica*), is inky-blue in color. It has a sweet, apple-like aroma.

Main Chemical Components of Essential Oil: Esters.

Main Therapeutic Properties of Essential Oil: Analgesic, antiseptic, antibacterial, anti-inflammatory, sedative, calming, emmenagogue.

Uses for Body Care: Oily skin, dry skin, eczema, dermatitis, acne.

Uses for Health: Arthritis, muscle pain, toothache, insomnia, stress, headache, back pain.

Uses for Women: Menopausal problems, cracked nipples, painful periods.

Uses for Babies and Children: Eczema, teething, insomnia.

Use for the Home: Shock, first-aid kit.

Use for Travel: Skin care, insect bites.

Social and Seasonal Use: Calming blends.

Ways to Use: Massage oils, diffusers, skin-care bases (scrubs, lotions, creams, butters, balms), sprays, bath products (oils, fizzes, melts, salts), candles. Also available as a hydrosol.

Cautions: May cause sensitivity in some people. Do not confuse with Moroccan chamomile (*Ormenis multicaulis*), which, although distantly related to both Roman chamomile and German chamomile, is not the same in chemical makeup.

Cost: $$

Cinnamon (Leaf)

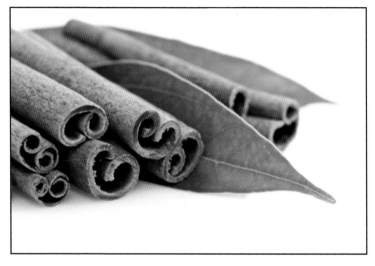

Botanical Name: *Cinnamomum zeylanicum.*

Synonyms: Cinnamon leaf, true cinnamon, *Cinnamomum verum.*

Botanical Family: *Lauraceae.*

Note: Base.

Blends Well with: Sweet orange, benzoin, clove (bud), spicy-oriental base note essential oils.

Alternative Oils: Clove (bud) (*Syzygium aromaticum*), basil (*Ocimum basilicum*).

Method of Extraction: Steam distillation of the leaves.

Distribution of Plant: Native to Sri Lanka and southern India, although there are many species of *Cinnamomum* available worldwide.

Description of Plant: A tropical, evergreen tree that grows up to forty-nine feet in height. It has small, white flowers, blue-white berries, and large, leathery leaves.

Characteristics of Essential Oil: Yellow-brown in color with a warm, spicy aroma.

Main Chemical Components of Essential Oil: Phenols.

Main Therapeutic Properties of Essential Oil: Antiseptic, astringent, aphrodisiac, digestive, astringent, emmenogogue.

Uses for Body Care: Warts.

Uses for Health: Poor circulation, rheumatism, diarrhea, colds, stress.

Uses for Women: Childbirth (under supervision); irregular, scant periods.

Uses for Babies and Children: Choose other essential oils in preference to cinnamon, due to chemical makeup.

Use for the Home: Cleaning.

Use for Travel: Diarrhea.

Social and Seasonal Use: Weddings, parties, winter blends.

Ways to Use: Massage oils, diffusers, skin-care bases (scrubs, lotions, creams, butters, balms), candles. Also available as a hydrosol.

Cautions: Avoid in pregnancy. It can cause irritation to the mucous membranes. Use in very low dilution and in moderation. Choose cinnamon leaf essential oil over cinnamon bark essential oil for therapeutic aromatherapy practice and in bath and body products. Cinnamon bark essential oil is a lot more toxic than cinnamon leaf essential oil.

Cost: $

Clary Sage

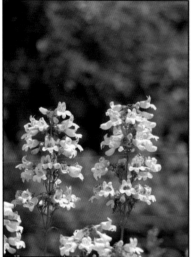

Botanical Name: *Salvia sclarea.*

Synonyms: Clary, clarry, eye bright, clear eye.

Botanical Family: *Lamiaceae.*

Note: Top.

Blends Well with: Lavender, geranium, citrus essential oils, cedarwood, peppermint.

Alternative Oils: True lavender (*Lavandula angustifolia*), Roman chamomile (*Chamaemelum nobile*).

Method of Extraction: Steam distillation of the flowers.

Distribution of Plant: Native to southern Europe. It is now found throughout the Mediterranean region, the United States, the United Kingdom, and various other countries.

Description of Plant: A perennial or biennial herb that grows up to approximately three feet in height. It has small purple-blue, mauve, or even pink flowers. It has a thick, hairy stem and long, green leaves.

Characteristics of Essential Oil: Pale or yellow-green in color with a sharp, herbaceaeous aroma.

Main Chemical Components of Essential Oil: Esters and alcohols.

Main Therapeutic Properties of Essential Oil: Antiseptic, antidepressant, aphrodisiac, antibacterial, astringent, emmenagogue, sedative, digestive.

Uses for Body Care: Oily skin, acne, mature skin, wrinkles.

Uses for Health: Muscle pain, asthma, depression, stress, panic attacks, hemorrhoids, flatulence.

Uses for Women: Postnatal depression, dysmenorrhea, menopausal problems, scant periods.

Uses for Babies and Children: Adolescence moodiness.

Use for the Home: Cleaning, air freshener.

Use for Travel: Minor digestive problems.

Social and Seasonal Use: Weddings, parties.

Ways to Use: Massage oils, diffusers, skin-care bases (scrubs, lotions, creams, butters, balms), sprays, candles. Also available as a hydrosol.

Cautions: Avoid use in pregnancy. Avoid using with alcohol as may induce a narcotic effect and increase drunkenness.

Cost: $

Clove (Bud)

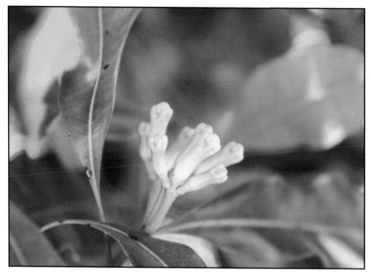

Botanical Name: *Syzygium aromaticum.*

Synonyms: *Eugenia caryophyllata, Eugenia carophyllus, Eugenia aromatica.*

Botanical Family: *Myrtaceae.*

Note: Base.

Blends Well with: Sweet orange, thyme, clary sage, rose, cinnamon (leaf), orange-based citrus oils.

Alternative Oils: Cinnamon (leaf) (*Cinnamomum zeylanicum*), basil (*Ocimum basilicum*).

Method of Extraction: Distillation of the clove buds.

Distribution of Plant: Possibly native to Indonesia. It is now cultivated in such places as Sri Lanka, India, the Philippines, Mauritius, and South America.

Description of Plant: An evergreen tree that grows up to thirty-nine feet in height. It has large, shiny leaves. The buds turn from pale green to deep red on maturity. The green buds produce a rosy-colored corolla, which then fades to bring forth a yellow-colored calyx—which finally matures to deep red. The calyx is then beaten from the tree and dried. The buds initially appear in the rainy season. The clove tree also has aromatic flowers.

Characteristics of Essential Oil: Pale yellow in color with a sweet and spicy aroma.

Main Chemical Components of Essential Oil: Phenols (namely, eugenol).

Main Therapeutic Properties of Essential Oil: Analgesic, antiseptic, anti-inflammatory, anti-infectious, antiviral, antibacterial, aphrodisiac, expectorant, mental stimulant.

Uses for Body Care: Acne.

Uses for Health: Toothache, wounds, sinusitis, rheumatoid arthritis, mental exhaustion, colds, flu.

Uses for Women: Uterine tonic: assists in childbirth, frigidity.

Uses for Babies and Children: Teething—use in dilution with a carrier oil and in minute quantities.

Use for the Home: Cleaning, air freshener, first-aid kit.

Use for Travel: Insect repellent.

Social and Seasonal Use: Winter blends, romantic blends, parties, celebrations, study aid.

Ways to Use: Massage oils, diffusers, skin-care bases (scrubs, lotions, creams, butters, balms), sprays, candles.

Cautions: Use in low dilution and in small quantities: risk of skin and mucous membrane irritation, if not used correctly. Use clove bud in preference to clove leaf essential oil for most therapeutic aromatherapy blends.

Cost: $

Cypress

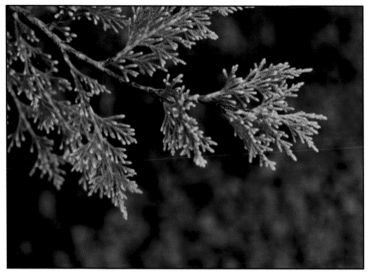

Botanical Name: *Cupressus sempervirens.*

Synonyms: Italian cypress, Mediterranean cypress, Graveyard cypress, Tucsan cypress.

Botanical Family: *Cupressaceae.*

Note: Base.

Blends Well with: Sweet orange, lavender, Roman chamomile, geranium, lemon, rose.

Alternative Oils: Juniper berry (*Juniperus communis*), black pepper (*Piper nigrum*).

Method of Extraction: Steam distillation of the needles and twigs.

Distribution of Plant: Native to the eastern Mediterranean region, Iran, Egypt, Israel, Syria, and various surrounding countries. It is found growing in countries such as France, Italy, Spain,

Portugal, and the United Kingdom, with various cultivars and species worldwide.

Description of Plant: An evergreen tree that is shaped like a cone. It has brown-colored cones, small flowers, and sprays of foliage. It grows to a height of 115 feet.

Characteristics of Essential Oil: Pale yellow to pale green in color. It has a woody, earthy, balsamic aroma, with spicy undertones.

Main Chemical Components of Essential Oil: Monoterpenes.

Main Therapeutic Properties of Essential Oil: Antiseptic, astringent, decongestant, antibacterial.

Uses for Body Care: Oily skin.

Uses for Health: Poor circulation, muscle cramps, asthma, bronchitis, irritability, stress.

Uses for Women: Menopausal problems, dysmenorrhea, PMS. excessive menstruation, irregular periods.

Uses for Babies and Children: Teenage skin problems, irritability.

Use for the Home: Cleaning, air freshener.

Use for Travel: Stress.

Social and Seasonal Use: Decongestant blends, winter blends, grief.

Ways to Use: Massage oils, diffusers, skin-care bases (scrubs, lotions, creams, butters, balms), sprays, bath products (oils, fizzes, melts, salts). Also available as a hydrosol.

Cautions: No known contraindications for general aromatherapy use.

Cost: $

Dill

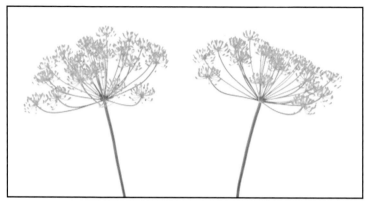

Botanical Name: *Anethum graveolens.*

Synonyms: *Peucedanum graveolens, Fractus Anethi,* dill weed (U.S.), dill seed.

Botanical Family: *Apiaceae.*

Note: Top.

Blends Well with: Lemon, spice essential oils.

Alternative Oils: Caraway (*Carum carvi*).

Method of Extraction: Distillation of the fresh, or dried, herb or seeds.

Distribution of Plant: Native to the Mediterranean region and the Black Sea area surrounding southern Russia. It is cultivated in many places, including Europe, the United States, and China.

Description of Plant: Annual or biennial herb that grows to a height of approximately two feet. It has umbels of yellow flowers and feather-like leaves. Dill has various chemeotypes. As a plant, it looks very similar to fennel (*Foeniculum vulgare*), although the chemical makeup of the two essential oils are completely different.

Characteristics of Essential Oil: Pale white to pale yellow in color with a warm, spicy aroma, similar to aniseed.

Main Chemical Components of Essential Oil: Ketones and monoterpenes.

Main Therapeutic Properties of Essential Oil: Antibacterial, digestive, sedative, antiseptic, emmenagogue, mucolytic.

Uses for Body Care: Wounds.

Uses for Health: Flatulence, indigestion, bronchitis.

Uses for Women: Lack of periods, assists childbirth, promotes milk production in nursing mothers.

Uses for Babies and Children: Traditionally used in dill water (an infusion of water and alcohol) for babies and children to remedy flatulence.

Use for the Home: Cleaning, first-aid kit.

Use for Travel: Minor digestive issues.

Social and Seasonal Use: Cleansing blends.

Ways to Use: Massage oils, diffusers, sprays. Also available as a hydrosol.

Cautions: Avoid in pregnancy.

Cost: $

Eucalyptus (Smithii)

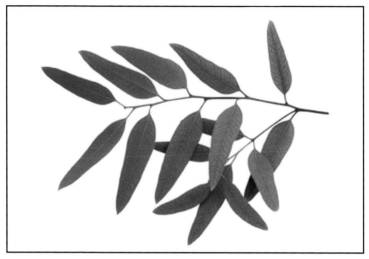

Botanical Name: *Eucalyptus Smithii.*
Synonyms: Eucalyptus, Gully gum.
Botanical Family: *Myrtaceae.*
Note: Top.
Blends Well with: Lemon, lavender, rosemary, peppermint, clove (bud).
Alternative Oils: Blue gum eucalyptus (*Eucalyptus* var. *globulus*).
Method of Extraction: Steam distillation of the leaves and twigs.
Distribution of Plant: Native to Australia but now also cultivated in southern Europe.
Description of Plant: A tall tree with pale green-gray leaves.
Characteristics of Essential Oil: Pale yellow in color with a sharp, camphoraceous aroma.
Main Chemical Components of Essential Oil: Oxides.

Main Therapeutic Properties of Essential Oil: Analgesic, antiseptic, antiviral, decongestant.

Uses for Body Care: Skin infections.

Uses for Health: Headaches, muscle pain, asthma, colds, flu, coughs.

Uses for Women: Headaches.

Uses for Babies and Children: A gentle oil for health issues.

Use for the Home: Cleaning, air freshener, laundry.

Use for Travel: Insect repellent.

Social and Seasonal Use: Cleaning yoga mat.

Ways to Use: Massage oils, diffusers, skin-care bases (scrubs, lotions, creams, butters, balms), sprays, candles.

Cautions: No known contraindications for general aromatherapy use. Do not confuse with lemon scented eucalyptus (*Eucalyptus citriodora*), eucalyptus dives (*Eucalyptus dives*), or eucalyptus staigeriana (*Eucalyptus staigeriana*), which contain differing chemical components from Eucalyptus smithii.

Cost: $

Fennel (Sweet)

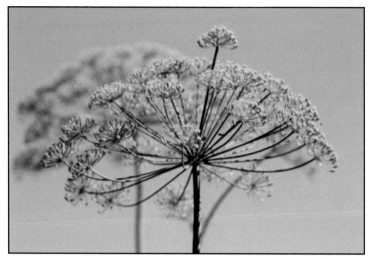

Botanical Name: *Foeniculum vulgare* var. *dulce.*

Synonyms: *Anethum foeniculum, Foeniculum vulgare, Foeniculum capillaceum,* sweet fennel, garden fennel, Roman fennel, French fennel.

Botanical Family: *Apiaceae.*

Note: Top to middle.

Blends Well with: Lemon, rose, myrrh, vetiver.

Alternative Oils: Thyme (*Thymus vulgaris* ct. thymol).

Method of Extraction: Steam distillation of the crushed seeds.

Distribution of Plant: Native to the Mediterranean region, including France, Greece, and Italy. It thrives particularly well in (non-windy) places near the ocean. It is now found throughout many countries of the world.

Description of Plant: Perennial or biennial herb that grows up to six feet tall. It blooms in mid to late summer with yellow umbels of flowers. It has fine, feathery foliage. As a plant, it looks very similar to dill (*Anethum graveolens*), although the chemical makeup of the two essential oils are completely different.

Characteristics of Essential Oil: Colorless to pale yellow in color with a sweet, aniseed aroma.

Main Chemical Components of Essential Oil: Phenols and monoterpenes.

Main Therapeutic Properties of Essential Oil: Anti-inflammatory, expectorant, antiseptic, emmenagogue, analgesic, antibacterial, decongestant, digestive.

Uses for Body Care: Oily skin, mature skin, wrinkles, bruises.

Uses for Health: Rheumatism, asthma, bronchitis, constipation, flatulence, indigestion, nausea.

Uses for Women: Amenorrhea, menopausal problems, assists childbirth, menstrual difficulties, stimulates milk production in nursing mothers.

Uses for Babies and Children: Not for use with babies and young children.

Use for the Home: Air fresheners, cleaning.

Use for Travel: Minor digestive issues.

Social and Seasonal Use: Cleansing blends.

Ways to Use: Massage oils, diffusers, skin-care bases (scrubs, lotions, creams, butters, balms), sprays, candles. Also available as a hydrosol.

Cautions: Avoid in pregnancy. Avoid with epilepsy. Do not use with babies and young children. Do not confuse with bitter fennel (*Foeniculum vulgare* var. *amarga*) essential oil, which contains a higher percentage of ketones in chemical makeup.

Cost: $

Frankincense

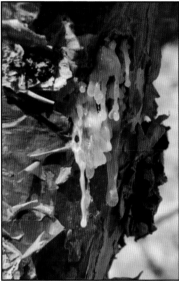

Botanical Name: *Boswellia carteri.*

Synonyms: Incense, olibanum, gum. The name literally translates as *high quality incense* from the Old French language *franc encens.*

Botanical Family: *Burseraceae.*

Note: Base.

Blends Well with: Rose, Roman chamomile, lavender, sandalwood, geranium, clary sage, vetiver, sweet orange, spice-based essential oils.

Alternative Oils: Scotch pine (*Pinus sylvestris*), black pepper (*Piper nigrum*), frankincense (*Boswellia frereana*), frankincense (*Boswellia sacra*).

Method of Extraction: Steam distillation of the gum resin. The resin exudes from the tree bark when it is cut. The tree has to reach maturity before it produces resin.

Distribution of Plant: Native to the Red Sea area of northeast Africa, although gum produced for frankincense essential oil is now available from places such as India, China, Oman (*Boswellia sacra*), and Somalia (*Boswellia frereana*).

Description of Plant: A small tree or shrub that produces white or pink flowers. It has green, pinnate leaves.

Characteristics of Essential Oil: Pale yellow in color with a predominant deep, spicy, balsamic aroma.

Main Chemical Components of Essential Oil: Monoterpenes.

Main Therapeutic Properties of Essential Oil: Antiseptic, anti-inflammatory, antidepressant, analgesic, astringent, sedative, expectorant, antibacterial, calming.

Uses for Body Care: Dry skin, mature skin, wrinkles.

Uses for Health: Anxiety, stress, depression, colds, asthma, bronchitis, slowing of breathing.

Uses for Women: Wrinkles, painful periods.

Uses for Babies and Children: Dry skin, expectorant, calming.

Use for the Home: First-aid kit.

Use for Travel: Dry skin.

Social and Seasonal Use: Yoga, weddings, parties, celebrations.

Ways to Use: Massage oils, diffusers, skin-care bases (scrubs, lotions, creams, butters, balms), perfume base, sprays, bath products (oils, fizzes, melts, salts), candles. Also available as a hydrosol.

Cautions: No known contraindications for general aromatherapy use. *Boswellia carteri* is listed as a threatened plant species, and consequently some aromatherapists are choosing to use alternative *Boswellia* species, including *Boswellia sacra* and *Boswellia frereana*. However, note that these species might not be the exact duplicate in chemical makeup.

Cost: $$

Geranium

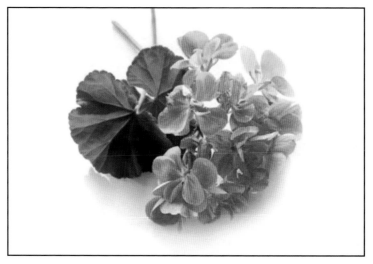

Botanical Name: *Pelargonium graveolens.*

Synonyms: Rose geranium, *Pelargonium*, Bourbon geranium.

Botanical Family: *Geraniaceae.*

Note: Middle.

Blends Well with: Rose, lavender, patchouli, floral essential oils, citrus essential oils, base note essential oils—such as sandalwood and cedarwood.

Alternative Oils: Rose (*Rosa damscena*), clary sage (*Salvia sclarea*), lavender (*Lavandula angustifolia*).

Method of Extraction: Steam distillation of the leaves and flowers.

Distribution of Plant: Native to South Africa but now cultivated worldwide in conducive climates. Reunion, France, and Egypt are popular places of essential oil production.

Description of Plant: An evergreen perennial plant that grows up to three feet in height. Both the leaves and the flowers are very aromatic. There are hundreds of species of geranium available, but the original color of the *Pelargonium* flowers is thought to be pink.

Characteristics of Essential Oil: Yellow-green in color, depending upon the area of production and species of cultivar. It has a sweet, rose-like aroma—although it is not as heady as the scent of rose.

Main Chemical Components of Essential Oil: Alcohols and esters.

Main Therapeutic Properties of Essential Oil: Anti-inflammatory, antiseptic, antibacterial, antiviral, astringent, decongestant, calming, analgesic, balancing.

Uses for Body Care: Mature skin, oily skin, acne, dermatitis, eczema.

Uses for Health: Stress, poor circulation, anxiety, hemorrhoids, rheumatism.

Uses for Women: Menstrual problems, menopausal problems, regulating hormone function, breast congestion, PMS.

Uses for Babies and Children: Teenage acne. Use in place of rose essential oil with babies.

Use for the Home: First-aid kit.

Use for Travel: Jet lag, insect bites.

Social and Seasonal Use: Weddings, parties, celebrations.

Ways to Use: Massage oils, diffusers, skin-care bases (scrubs, lotions, creams, butters, balms), perfume base, sprays, bath products (oils, fizzes, melts, salts), candles. Also available as a hydrosol.

Cautions: No known contraindications for general aromatherapy use. Some species of geranium (for example, Bourbon) may cause skin sensitivity.

Cost: $

Ginger

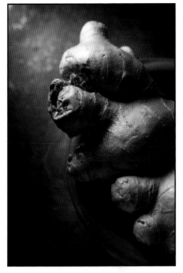

Botanical Name: *Zingiber officinale.*
Synonyms: Common ginger, Jamaica ginger, ginger root.
Botanical Family: *Zingiberaceae.*
Note: Top.
Blends Well with: Rose, sweet orange, cinnamon, vetiver, lime, lemon, frankincense, cedarwood.
Alternative Oils: Cedarwood (*Cedrus atlantica*).
Method of Extraction: Steam distillation of the unpeeled, dried, ground rhizome (root).
Distribution of Plant: Native to Southern Asia but now cultivated in the Caribbean (including Jamaica), East Africa, Japan, India, and China.

Description of Plant: A perennial herb that grows up to three feet in height. It has white or pink buds that blossom into yellow flowers. However, it is the rhizome root below ground that is aromatic.

Characteristics of Essential Oil: Pale yellow or amber in color with a deep, warm, spicy aroma.

Main Chemical Components of Essential Oil: Sesquiterpenes, monoterpenes, and alcohols.

Main Therapeutic Properties of Essential Oil: Analgesic, antiseptic, aphrodisiac, antibacterial, carminative, expectorant, digestive.

Uses for Body Care: High concentrations of ginger essential oil can irritate the skin in skin-care products; use with caution.

Uses for Health: Arthritis, muscle pain, fatigue, poor circulation, rheumatism, coughs, flatulence, diarrhea, indigestion, nausea, sinusitis, bronchitis, colds.

Uses for Women: Morning sickness.

Uses for Babies and Children: Nausea, digestive.

Use for the Home: First-aid kit.

Use for Travel: Travel sickness, nausea, minor stomach upsets.

Social and Seasonal Use: Grounding blends, parties, celebrations.

Ways to Use: Massage oils, diffusers, skin-care bases (scrubs, lotions, creams, butters, balms), sprays, candles. Also available as a hydrosol.

Cautions: Use in moderation to avoid skin sensitization: possibly slightly phototoxic.

Cost: $

Grapefruit

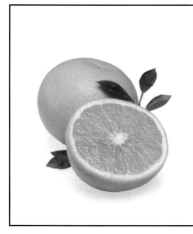

Botanical Name: *Citrus x paradisi.*
Synonyms: Shaddock, *Citrus maxima* var. *racemose*, *Citrus racemosa*, Chakotra (Hindi).
Botanical Family: *Rutaceae.*
Note: Top.
Blends Well with: Lemon, cypress, geranium, lavender.
Alternative Oils: Lemon (*Citrus limon*), mandarin (*Citrus reticulata*), sweet orange (*Citrus sinensis*).

Method of Extraction: Cold expression of the fresh rind or peel.

Distribution of Plant: Native to tropical Asia and the West Indies. It is cultivated predominantly in California, Florida, and Brazil. The grapefruit is a hybrid that was the result of a cross-pollination between the shaddock or pomelo (*Citrus maxima*) and the sweet orange (*Citrus sinensis*). The verifiable history of its hybridization is not clearly documented, but it is believed to have originated some time in the eighteenth century.

Description of Plant: A cultivated tree that grows to a height of thirty-three feet. It has shiny, green leaves and star-shaped, white flowers. The flowers are aromatic. However, it is the large, yellow fruits that the essential oil is extracted from.

Characteristics of Essential Oil: Yellow or pale green in color with a sweet, citrus aroma.

Main Chemical Components of Essential Oil: Monoterpenes (namely, limonene).

Main Therapeutic Properties of Essential Oil: Antiseptic, anti-bacterial, digestive, astringent, antiviral, diuretic, calming.

Uses for Body Care: Oily skin, acne.

Uses for Health: Colds, flu, water retention, stress, depression, headaches.

Uses for Women: Cellulitis.

Uses for Babies and Children: Gentle and uplifting: a "happy" oil for children.

Use for the Home: Air fresheners, cleaning.

Use for Travel: Jet lag, minor stomach upsets.

Social and Seasonal Use: Use to improve concentration levels for work and study, and in blends for conversation starters/social mingling at parties.

Ways to Use: Massage oils, diffusers, skin-care bases (scrubs, lotions, creams, butters, balms), sprays, bath products (oils, fizzes, melts, salts), candles. Also available as a hydrosol.

Cautions: No known contraindications for general aromatherapy use. Unlike many citrus essential oils, it is not known to be photo-toxic. However, it has a short shelf life and is quick to oxidize.

Cost: $

Helichrysum

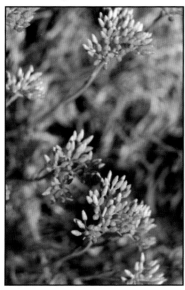

Botanical Name: *Helichrysum angustifolium.*

Synonyms: Everlasting, *Immortelle, Helichrysum italicum*, curry plant.

Botanical Family: *Asteraceae.*

Note: Base.

Blends Well with: Geranium, rose, lavender, citrus essential oils.

Alternative Oils: Lavender (*Lavandula angustifolia*).

Method of Extraction: Steam distillation of the fresh flowers.

Distribution of Plant: Native to the Mediterranean region and north Africa. It is now cultivated in many countries, depending upon species and subspecies.

Description of Plant: An aromatic herb that grows up to two feet in height. It has bright yellow, daisy-like flowers, a characteristic of the *Asteraceae* plant family. It has narrow, silver-colored leaves. The flowers still retain their yellow color, even as they dry out.

Characteristics of Essential Oil: Pale yellow to red in color. It has a rich, honey-like aroma.

Main Chemical Components of Essential Oil: Alcohols and esters.

Main Therapeutic Properties of Essential Oil: Anti-inflammatory, antimicrobial, antiseptic, astringent, cicatrizant, expectorant.

Uses for Body Care: Dry skin, acne, eczema, dermatitis.

Uses for Health: Inflammation, wound healing, cuts, burns, muscle pain, rheumatism, asthma, bronchitis, colds, flu, depression, stress.

Uses for Women: Skin care.

Uses for Babies and Children: Cuts, wounds.

Use for the Home: First-aid kit.

Use for Travel: Sunburn, insect bites.

Social and Seasonal Use: Weddings, parties, celebrations.

Ways to Use: Massage oils, diffusers, skin-care bases (scrubs, lotions, creams, butters, balms), perfume base, sprays, bath products (oils, fizzes, melts, salts), candles. Also available as a hydrosol.

Cautions: No known contraindications for general aromatherapy use.

Cost: $$$

Jasmine

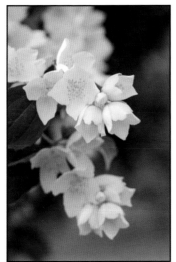

Botanical Name: *Jasminum officinale.*

Synonyms: *Jasmine Grandiflorum*, common jasmine, jessamine, jasmin, "king of flowers."

Botanical Family: *Oleaceae.*

Note: Base.

Blends Well with: Geranium, sandalwood, cedarwood, citrus essential oils.

Alternative Oils: Neroli (*Citrus aurantium* var. *amara*), clary sage (*Salvia sclarea*), lavender (*Lavandula angustifolia*).

Method of Extraction: A concrete is solvent extracted (from the flowers) to produce jasmine absolute.

Distribution of Plant: Native to west Asia, northern India, and China, depending upon species and/or cultivar. There are many varieties of jasmine, and sometimes two species are so closely related that they are treated as one and the same variety.

Description of Plant: An evergreen shrub that can climb or grow to lengths or heights of up to thirty-three feet (depending upon exact species). It has star-shaped, white flowers that are highly aromatic. The leaves are green and pinnate.

Characteristics of Essential Oil: A viscous, dark brown or orange colored absolute, with a rich, heady, floral aroma.

Main Chemical Components of Essential Oil: Esters and alcohols.

Main Therapeutic Properties of Essential Oil: Antidepressant, anti-inflammatory, antiseptic, aphrodisiac, sedative, expectorant, uterine tonic, mild analgesic.

Uses for Body Care: Dry skin, sensitive skin.

Uses for Health: Depression, stress, coughs, muscular spasms.

Uses for Women: Dysmenorrhea, labor pain, stretch marks, stimulates childbirth (uterine contractions), stimulates milk production.

Uses for Babies and Children: Jasmine is an absolute and not a pure essential oil. Choose alternative essential oils over jasmine.

Use for the Home: Shock, accidents, and bereavements; jasmine helps to regulate breathing.

Use for Travel: Sensitive skin protection.

Social and Seasonal Use: Weddings, parties, celebrations.

Ways to Use: Massage oils, diffusers, skin-care bases (scrubs, lotions, creams, butters, balms), perfume base, sprays, bath products (oils, fizzes, melts, salts), candles.

Cautions: No known contraindications for general aromatherapy use. However, it is advisable to avoid use in pregnancy as jasmine may stimulate uterine contractions. Be aware that there are various species of jasmine available as an absolute, for example, *Jasminum sambac*.

Cost: $$$

Juniper (Berry)

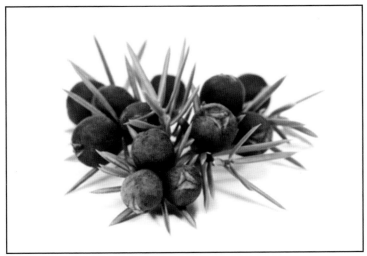

Botanical Name: *Juniperus communis.*

Synonyms: Common juniper.

Botanical Family: *Cupressaceae.*

Note: Middle.

Blends Well with: Sweet orange, lavender, geranium, vetiver, cedarwood, black pepper.

Alternative Oils: Cypress (*Cupressus sempervirens*), silver fir (*Abies alba*), Scotch pine (*Pinus sylvestris*).

Method of Extraction: Steam distillation of the berries.

Distribution of Plant: Native to Scandinavia, northern Europe, Canada, Siberia, and northern Asia.

Description of Plant: An evergreen tree that grows up to a height of twenty feet. It has green needles, small flowers, and green berries. The berries turn black in color on maturity.

Characteristics of Essential Oil: White to pale yellow in color, with a woody-balsamic aroma and a green top note.

Main Chemical Components of Essential Oil: Monoterpenes.

Main Therapeutic Properties of Essential Oil: Antiseptic, aphrodisiac, astringent, cicatrizant, sedative, emmenagogue, diuretic, expectorant, detoxifying.

Uses for Body Care: Oily skin, acne, eczema, dermatitis.

Uses for Health: Rheumatism, colds, flu, anxiety, stress, bronchitis, gout, fluid retention.

Uses for Women: Dysmennorrhea, menstrual problems, uterine stimulant.

Uses for Babies and Children: Avoid in use with babies and children.

Use for the Home: Air fresheners, cleaning.

Use for Travel: Skin conditions.

Social and Seasonal Use: Weddings, parties, celebrations.

Ways to Use: Massage oils, diffusers, skin-care bases (scrubs, lotions, creams, butters, balms), perfume base, sprays, bath products (oils, fizzes, melts, salts), candles. Also available as a hydrosol.

Cautions: Avoid use in pregnancy as it may stimulate the uterine muscle. In addition, avoid if you have kidney disease. There is also an essential oil distilled from the needles and twigs of the juniper tree.

Cost: $

Lavender (True)

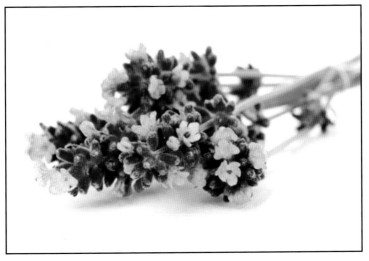

Botanical Name: *Lavandula officinalis, Lavandula angustifolia, Lavandula vera.*

Synonyms: Common lavender, true lavender, garden lavender.

Botanical Family: *Lamiaceae.*

Note: Middle.

Blends Well with: Floral, citrus, and spice oils.

Alternative Oils: Spike lavender (*Lavandula latifolia*), lavandin (*Lavandula x intermedia*).

Method of Extraction: Steam distillation of the flowers.

Distribution of Plant: Native to the Mediterranean region, but it is now found in nearly all corners of the world. Both French and English lavender species are thought to produce some of the best essential oils.

Description of Plant: An evergreen herb with violet-blue flowers in the spring and summer. It grows up to three feet in height.

It has narrow, linear leaves with flowers on the spikes. True lavender only grows at or above altitudes of 2,000 feet.

Characteristics of Essential Oil: Colorless to pale yellow in color. It has a sweet, floral aroma with a woody undertone.

Main Chemical Components of Essential Oil: Alcohols and esters; percentage varies depending upon species and chemotype.

Main Therapeutic Properties of Essential Oil: Analgesic, antibacterial, antidepressant, antifunga, anti-inflammatory, antiseptic, cicatrizant, emmenagogue, insecticide, sedative, stimulant.

Uses for Body Care: Dry skin, oily skin, nail care, eczema, dermatitis, acne.

Uses for Health: Stress, wounds, headaches, burns, muscular aches and pains, insomnia, depression.

Uses for Women: Pregnancy, stretch marks, labor, cracked nipples.

Uses for Babies and Children: Insomnia, abdominal pain, eczema, insect bites, chicken pox, sunburn, wounds.

Use for the Home: Air freshener, washing down kitchen and bathroom surfaces, moth repellent, sachets, first-aid kit.

Use for Travel: Jet lag (relaxant), sunburn, insect bites.

Social and Seasonal Use: Weddings, parties.

Ways to Use: Massage oils, diffusers, skin-care bases (scrubs, lotions, creams, butters, balms), perfume base, sprays, bath products (oils, fizzes, melts, salts), candles. Also available as a hydrosol.

Cautions: One of the most used essential oils. Gentle, non-sensitizing and non-irritating in the majority of cases.

Cost: $

Lemon

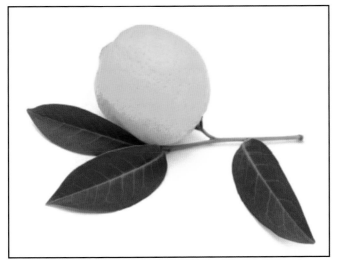

Botanical Name: *Citrus limon.*

Synonyms: *Citrus limonum,* Cedro oil, citron.

Botanical Family: *Rutaceae.*

Note: Top.

Blends Well with: Other citrus essential oils, lavender, geranium, spicy and floral base note essential oils.

Alternative Oils: Lime (*Citrus aurantifolia*), sweet orange (*Citrus sinensis*).

Method of Extraction: Cold expression of the outer, fresh peel of the fruit.

Distribution of Plant: Native to Asia—although it is now common throughout the Mediterranean region, California, Florida, Cyprus, Italy, and other areas of the world with warm, sunny climates.

Description of Plant: An evergreen fruit tree that grows up to twenty feet in height. It has oval, green leaves and fragrant flowers. It has sharp thorns that distinguish it from other fruit trees. The yellow-colored fruit is about the size and shape of an egg, but can vary.

Characteristics of Essential Oil: Pale green to yellow in color, with a light, green, citrus aroma.

Main Chemical Components of Essential Oil: Monoterpenes.

Main Therapeutic Properties of Essential Oil: Antibacterial, antimicrobial, antiviral, anti-infectious, astringent, digestive.

Uses for Body Care: Oily skin, dry skin, mature skin, acne.

Uses for Health: Poor circulation, colds, flu, digestive complaints, asthma.

Uses for Women: Cellulite.

Uses for Babies and Children: Lack of confidence, clinginess.

Use for the Home: Air fresheners, cleaning, first-aid kit.

Use for Travel: Minor stomach upsets.

Social and Seasonal Use: Concentration and mood at work, cleaning yoga mat, conversation starters/social mingling for parties, uplifting blends.

Ways to Use: Massage oils, diffusers, skin-care bases (scrubs, lotions, creams, butters, balms), sprays, bath products (oils, fizzes, melts, salts), candles.

Cautions: Phototoxic. Avoid use in sunlight, prior to going out in sunlight, or with the use of other ultraviolet sources such as tanning units. Possible skin sensitization.

Cost: $

Lime

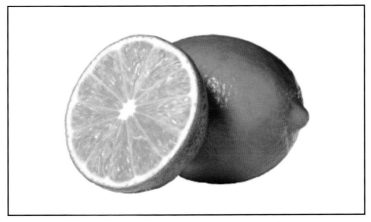

Botanical Name: *Citrus aurantifolia.*

Synonyms: Key lime, West Indian lime, Mexican lime, bartender's lime, *Citrus medica* var. *acida, Citrus latifolia*—Persian lime, Tahiti lime.

Botanical Family: *Rutaceae.*

Note: Top.

Blends Well with: Other citrus essential oils, lavender, citronella, neroli.

Alternative Oils: Lemon (*Citrus limon*), sweet orange (*Citrus sinensis*).

Method of Extraction: Expressed lime essential oil by cold expression of the outer, fresh peel of the fruit. Distilled lime essential oil is also available from the crushing of the whole fruit (a by-product of the juice industry).

Distribution of Plant: Naturalized in most tropical and subtropical regions of the world, including Mexico, Italy, and Florida. It is thought to be of south Asian origin.

Description of Plant: A small, evergreen tree that grows up to fifteen feet in height. The tree has sharp spines, ovate leaves, and small, white flowers. The fruit, which is about half the size of lemon (depending upon species), is pale green in color.

Characteristics of Essential Oil: Pale yellow to olive-green in color with a sharp, citrus aroma. The expressed essential oil is sweeter in aroma than the distilled essential oil.

Main Chemical Components of Essential Oil: Monoterpenes. The distilled essential oil contains only traces of coumarins, unlike the expressed essential oil.

Main Therapeutic Properties of Essential Oil: Antiseptic, antiviral, antibacterial, tonic.

Uses for Body Care: oily skin, acne, brittle nails.

Uses for Health: Poor circulation, colds, flu, digestive complaints, asthma, high blood pressure.

Uses for Women: Cellulite.

Uses for Babies and Children: Use in place of lemon essential oil.

Use for the Home: Air fresheners, cleaning, first-aid kit.

Use for Travel: Minor stomach upsets.

Social and Seasonal Use: Concentration and mood at work, cleaning yoga mat, conversation starters/social mingling for parties, uplifting blends.

Ways to Use: Massage oils, diffusers, skin-care bases (scrubs, lotions, creams, butters, balms), sprays, bath products (oils, fizzes, melts, salts), candles.

Cautions: The expressed essential oil is phototoxic. Avoid use in sunlight, prior to going out in sunlight, or with the use of other ultraviolet sources such as tanning units. The distilled essential oil is non-phototoxic.

Cost: $

Marjoram (Sweet)

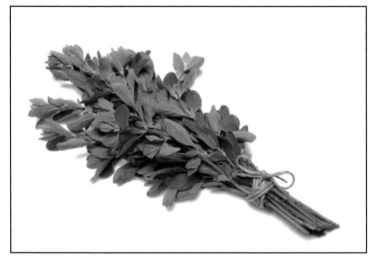

Botanical Name: *Origanum marjorana.*

Synonyms: *Marjorana hortensis*, knotted marjoram.

Botanical Family: *Lamiaceae.*

Note: Middle.

Blends Well with: Lavender, geranium,cypress, eucalyptus, black pepper, cedarwood, "orange-based" citrus essential oils.

Alternative Oils: Neroli (*Citrus aurantium* var. *amara*), rose (*Rosa damascena*), tea tree (*Melaleuca alternifolia*).

Method of Extraction: Steam distillation of the flowering herb (dried).

Distribution of Plant: Native to the Mediterranean region and north Africa, including Portugal and Egypt. It is now cultivated in many countries, including the United States.

Description of Plant: A perennial, or annual, herb (depending upon climate) that grows up to two feet in height. It has green, oval leaves and small, white flowers. The whole plant is fragrant.

Characteristics of Essential Oil: Pale yellow to amber in color. It has a warm, spicy aroma with camphoraceous overtones.

Main Chemical Components of Essential Oil: Alcohols and monoterpenes.

Main Therapeutic Properties of Essential Oil: Analgesic, antiseptic, antiviral, antibacterial, anti-infectious, expectorant, sedative, emmenagogue.

Uses for Body Care: Bruises.

Uses for Health: Arthritis, muscle pain, asthma, bronchitis, insomnia, stress, depression, headaches, respiratory complaints.

Uses for Women: Painful periods, PMS, amenorrhea.

Uses for Babies and Children: Chest infections.

Use for the Home: Air fresheners, cleaning.

Use for Travel: Respiratory problems, headaches, insomnia.

Social and Seasonal Use: Weddings (herbs, such as marjoram, were traditional in Greek and Roman bridal crowns), romantic blends (marjoram is a traditional ingredient in love potions).

Ways to Use: Massage oils, diffusers, skin-care bases (scrubs, lotions, creams, butters, balms), sprays, bath products (oils, fizzes, melts, salts), candles.

Cautions: Avoid during pregnancy. Do not confuse sweet marjoram (*Origanum marjorana*) with common oregano (*Origanum vulgare*), which is sometimes referred to as marjoram. In addition, Spanish marjoram (*Thymus mastichina*) is not the same as sweet marjoram. Both common oregano and Spanish marjoram are made up of different chemical components from sweet marjoram.

Cost: $

Melissa

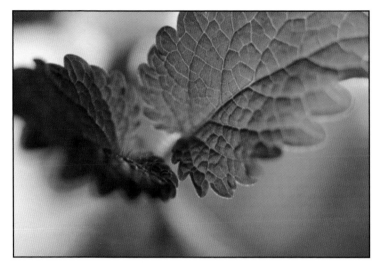

Botanical Name: *Melissa officinalis.*

Synonyms: Lemon balm, sweet balm, heart's delight, common balm, bee balm (although not to be confused with Mondara *sp.* (bergamot)).

Botanical Family: *Lamiaceae.*

Note: Middle.

Blends Well with: Floral and citrus essential oils, especially rose, geranium, lavender, bergamot.

Alternative Oils: Lemongrass (*Cymbopogon citratus*), lemon scented eucalyptus (*Eucalyptus citriodora*).

Method of Extraction: Steam distillation of the leaves and flowers.

Distribution of Plant: Native to the Mediterranean region but now also cultivated in north Africa, the United States, the United Kingdom, and various other places.

Description of Plant: A small, perennial herb that grows up to two feet in height. It has green, ovate, serrated leaves that are fragrant when rubbed. It also has small, white flowers that attract bees (from which melissa takes its English name: *Melissa* means *honey bee* in the Greek language).

Characteristics of Essential Oil: Yellow in color with a sweet, fresh, lemon aroma, with minty undertones.

Main Chemical Components of Essential Oil: Aldehydes.

Main Therapeutic Properties of Essential Oil: Antidepressant, antibacterial, sedative, uterine tonic, emmenogogue, sedative.

Uses for Body Care: All types of skin-care, eczema.

Uses for Health: Asthma, bronchitis, nausea, anxiety, depression, indigestion, migraine.

Uses for Women: Menstrual problems, menopausal problems.

Uses for Babies and Children: Infections.

Use for the Home: Air fresheners, shock.

Use for Travel: Insect bites, insect repellent.

Social and Seasonal Use: Weddings, parties, celebrations.

Ways to Use: Massage oils, diffusers, skin-care bases (scrubs, lotions, creams, butters, balms), sprays, candles. Also available as a hydrosol.

Cautions: Avoid during pregnancy. Melissa essential oil may cause skin irritation, so use in low dilution and in moderation. Melissa essential oil is also frequently adulterated due to its high cost; be careful that the oil has not been diluted with other essential oils such as lemon (*Citrus limon*) and lemongrass (*Cymbopogon citratus*), which have a strong, lemon aroma.

Cost: $$$

Myrrh

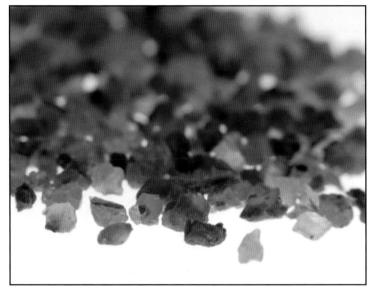

Botanical Name: *Commiphora myrrha.*

Synonyms: Common myrrh, gum myrrh, *Balsamodendron myrrha*, *Commiphora myrrha* var. *molmol*, hirabol myrrh.

Botanical Family: *Burseraceae.*

Note: Base.

Blends Well with: Frankincense, sweet orange, mandarin, lavender, benzoin, sandalwood, spice essential oils.

Alternative Oils: Patchouli (*Pogostemon cablin*).

Method of Extraction: Steam distillation of the crude myrrh. Solvent extraction of the crude myrrh produces a myrrh resinoid.

Distribution of Plant: Native to southwest Asia and northeast Africa.

Description of Plant: A shrub or small tree that grows up to thirty-three feet in height. It has knotted branches, white flowers, and fragrant leaves. When the tissue between ducts in the bark of the tree breaks down, it forms cavities. These cavities become filled with a crude myrrh secretion that naturally discharges from the bark or when the bark is cut. The initial substance is fluid but hardens to a brittle mass that is red-brown in color.

Characteristics of Essential Oil: Yellow in color with a balsamic, medicinal aroma. The resinoid is red-brown in color with a spicy, balsamic aroma; it is solid at room temperature.

Main Chemical Components of Essential Oil: Alcohols and sesquiterpenes.

Main Therapeutic Properties of Essential Oil: Anti-inflammatory, antiseptic, antimicrobial, antifunga, astringent, cicatrizant, emmenagogue, expectorant, sedative.

Uses for Body Care: Cracked skin, mature skin, wrinkles, eczema.

Uses for Health: Arthritis, wounds, asthma, coughs, colds, flatulence, hemorrhoids, athlete's foot.

Uses for Women: Amenorrhea.

Uses for Babies and Children: skin-care.

Use for the Home: Air fresheners.

Use for Travel: Wounds, skin-care.

Social and Seasonal Use: Weddings, parties and celebrations, relaxing blends, Christmas blends.

Ways to Use: Massage oils, diffusers, skin-care bases (scrubs, lotions, creams, butters, balms), perfume base, sprays, bath products (oils, fizzes, melts, salts), candles. Also available as a hydrosol.

Cautions: Avoid during pregnancy.

Cost: $$

Myrtle

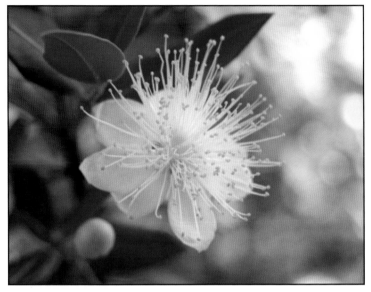

Botanical Name: *Myrtus communis.*

Synonyms: Corsican pepper (*poivrier corse* in the French language), common myrtle, true myrtle.

Botanical Family: *Myrtaceae.*

Note: Top to middle.

Blends Well with: Eucalyptus, lavender, cedarwood, pine, spice essential oils.

Alternative Oils: Niaouli (*Melaleuca viridiflora*), eucalyptus smithii (*Eucalyptus smithii*), spike lavender (*Lavandula latifolia*).

Method of Extraction: Steam distillation of the leaves and twigs.

Distribution of Plant: Native to north Africa. It is now found growing wild throughout Europe.

Description of Plant: A large bush or small tree that grows up to fifteen feet in height, depending on cultivar. It has a bark that is red-brown in color; green, pointed leaves; and white flowers. Both the flowers and the leaves are aromatic. The flowers are followed by black berries.

Characteristics of Essential Oil: Pale yellow in color with a fresh, camphoraceous aroma with slight woody-spicy undertones. Not dissimilar to eucalyptus in aroma, although more woody-spicy.

Main Chemical Components of Essential Oil: Oxides, alcohols, and monoterpenes.

Main Therapeutic Properties of Essential Oil: Antiseptic, astringent, antibacterial, expectorant, balsamic, immuno-stimulant.

Uses for Body Care: Oily skin, acne.

Uses for Health: Asthma, bronchitis, colds, flu, hemorrhoids, rheumatism, arthritis.

Uses for Women: skin-care.

Uses for Babies and Children: Choose another essential oil in preference.

Use for the Home: Air fresheners.

Use for Travel: Choose another essential oil in preference.

Social and Seasonal Use: Cleansing blends.

Ways to Use: Massage oils, diffusers, skin-care bases (scrubs, lotions, creams, butters, balms), sprays, candles. Also available as a hydrosol.

Cautions: No known contraindications for general aromatherapy use.

Cost: $

Neroli

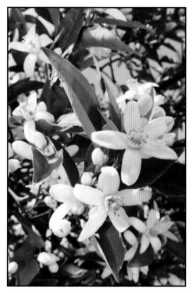

Botanical Name: *Citrus auran-tium* var. *amara.*

Synonyms: Orange blossom, orange flower, neroli biga-rade, *Citrus Bigaradia*, *Citrus aurantium* var. *amara flos.*

Botanical Family: *Rutaceae.*

Note: Base.

Blends Well with: Sweet orange, lavender, geranium, clary sage, rose, citrus essen-tial oils.

Alternative Oils: Petitgrain (*Citrus aurantium* var. *amara*), petitgrain sur fleurs/petit-grain neroli (a distilled blend of both neroil and petitgrain essential oils).

Method of Extraction: Steam distillation of the fresh flowers. It is also possible to produce an absolute through solvent extraction.

Distribution of Plant: Native to the Far East. Today, it is grown in the Mediterranean region, United States, and north Africa.

Description of Plant: An evergreen tree that grows up to thirty-three feet in height. It has glossy, green leaves. The white flowers are aromatic. Neroli essential oil is distilled from the bitter orange tree, which also produces petitgrain essential oil (from the leaves) and bitter orange essential oil (from the fruit).

Characteristics of Essential Oil: Pale yellow in color. It has a deep, intoxicating, floral aroma, with citrus orange overtones.

Main Chemical Components of Essential Oil: Alcohols, mono-terpenes, and esters.

Main Therapeutic Properties of Essential Oil: Antiseptic, anti-depressant, aphrodisiac, antibacterial, digestive, calming.

Uses for Body Care: Sensitive skin, mature skin, wrinkles.

Uses for Health: Anxiety, stress, depression, fatigue, insomnia, hemorrhoids, flatulence, lowers blood pressure, poor circulation.

Uses for Women: PMS, menopausal problems, varicose veins.

Uses for Babies and Children: Gentle to use in skin-care and anxiety.

Use for the Home: Shock.

Use for Travel: Fatigue, skin-care, stress.

Social and Seasonal Use: Weddings (sprigs of neroli used to be woven into European bridal crowns to ease a bride's wedding day nerves), parties, celebrations, romantic blends.

Ways to Use: Massage oils, diffusers, skin-care bases (scrubs, lotions, creams, butters, balms), perfume base, sprays, bath products (oils, fizzes, melts, salts), candles. Also available as a hydrosol.

Cautions: No known contraindications for general aromatherapy use. The flowers of the sweet orange (*Citrus sinensis*) tree are also distilled and sold as neroli (*Neroli petalae*) essential oil; however, this essential oil is of a lesser quality than a true neroli essential oil distillate made from the flowers of the bitter orange tree.

Cost: $$$

Orange (Sweet)

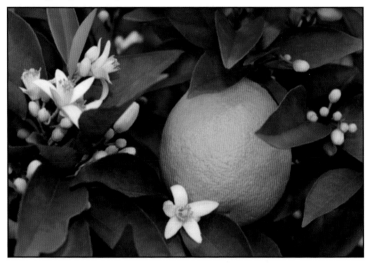

Botanical Name: *Citrus sinensis.*

Synonyms: *Citrus aurantium* var. *sinensis, Citrus aurantium* var. *dulcis,* Citrus bigarde, Seville orange, Portugal orange.

Botanical Family: *Rutaceae.*

Note: Top.

Blends Well with: Neroli, lavender, rose, ginger, clove, cypress, cedarwood, frankincense, myrrh, spice essential oils.

Alternative Oils: Bitter orange (*Citrus aurantium* var. *amara*), mandarin (*Citrus reticulata*), grapefruit (*Citrus paradisi*).

Method of Extraction: Cold expression or steam distillation of the fresh, outer peel.

Distribution of Plant: Native to China but prevalent in many countries of the world today, including the Mediterranean region, United States (California, Florida), and Brazil.

Description of Plant: An evergreen tree that is similar in appearance to the bitter orange tree but is more sensitive to colder weather. It has dark green leaves and few spines. The fruit, which is orange in color, is larger and paler in color than the bitter orange variety.

Characteristics of Essential Oil: Yellow-amber or orange in color. It has a fresh, light, fruity aroma.

Main Chemical Components of Essential Oil: Monoterpenes.

Main Therapeutic Properties of Essential Oil: Antidepressant, anti-inflammatory, antiseptic, antibacterial, digestive, sedative.

Uses for Body Care: Oily skin.

Uses for Health: Constipation, diarrhea, digestive problems, colds, flu, stress.

Uses for Women: Varicose veins.

Uses for Babies and Children: Digestive problems, travel sickness, "happy" oil for children.

Use for the Home: Air fresheners.

Use for Travel: Travel sickness, minor digestive problems.

Social and Seasonal Use: Conversation starters/social mingling at parties and celebrations, at work (mood uplifter).

Ways to Use: Massage oils, diffusers, skin-care bases (scrubs, lotions, creams, butters, balms), sprays, bath products (oils, fizzes, melts, salts), candles.

Cautions: No known contraindications for general aromatherapy use. However, distilled sweet orange essential oil is phototoxic, whereas expressed sweet orange oil is not phototoxic. Distilled sweet orange essential oil oxidizes quickly. There is a risk of possible skin sensitization in some people.

Cost: $

Patchouli

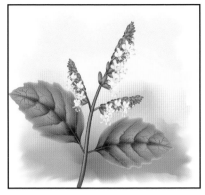

Botanical Name: *Pogestemon cablin.*

Synonyms: Patchouly, pachouli, puchaput, puchapat, *Pogestomon patchouly.*

Botanical Family: *Lamiaceae.*

Note: Base.

Blends Well with: Sweet orange, lavender, rose, neroli, geranium, most base note and spice essential oils.

Alternative Oils: Myrrh (*Commihora myrrha*).

Method of Extraction: Steam distillation of the dried (fermented) leaves.

Distribution of Plant: Native to Indonesia and the Philippines. It is now cultivated in countries and continents with a similar climate, for example, South America.

Description of Plant: A perennial herb that grows up to three feet in height. It has large, fragrant leaves with purple-white flowers.

Characteristics of Essential Oil: Amber or dark orange in color. The essential oil is thick and viscous in nature. It has a rich, sickly-sweet, earthy aroma that actually improves with age.

Main Chemical Components of Essential Oil: Sesquiterpenes and alcohols.

Main Therapeutic Properties of Essential Oil: Anti-inflammatory, antimicrobial, antiseptic, antiviral, aphrodisiac, astringent, cicatrizant, balancing, and calming.

Uses for Body Care: Cracked skin, oily skin, acne, wrinkles, eczema, dermatitis.

Uses for Health: Wounds, stress, hair care, depression, hemorrhoids.

Uses for Women: Varicose veins.

Uses for Babies and Children: skin-care.

Use for the Home: Choose other essential oils in preference.

Use for Travel: Insect repellent.

Social and Seasonal Use: Yoga, weddings, parties.

Ways to Use: Massage oils, diffusers, skin-care bases (scrubs, lotions, creams, butters, balms), perfume base, sprays, bath products (oils, fizzes, melts, salts), candles. Also available as a hydrosol.

Cautions: No known contraindications for general aromatherapy use.

Cost: $

Pepper (Black)

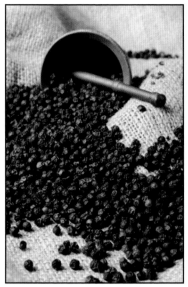

Botanical Name: *Piper nigrum.*
Synonyms: Pepper, piper.
Botanical Family: *Piperaceae.*
Note: Middle.
Blends Well with: Sweet orange, clove, cinnamon, lavender, frankincense, lemon.
Alternative Oils: Juniper berry (*Juniperus communis*), nutmeg (*Myristica fragrans*), yarrow (*Achillea millefolium*).
Method of Extraction: Steam distillation of the dried, crushed peppercorns/berries.
Distribution of Plant: Native to India and China. It is now cultivated in Malaysia, Indonesia, and other locales with a similar climate.
Description of Plant: A perennial woody vine with heart-shaped leaves and small, white flowers. It grows between sixteen and twenty feet in length. It has small, red berries that turn to black on maturity.
Characteristics of Essential Oil: White to pale green in color. It has a warm, woody, spicy aroma.
Main Chemical Components of Essential Oil: Monoterpenes and sesquiterpenes.
Main Therapeutic Properties of Essential Oil: Analgesic, antiseptic, digestive, expectorant, aphrodisiac, antibacterial.
Uses for Body Care: Chilblains.

Uses for Health: Bronchitis, rheumatism, arthritis, muscle pain, poor circulation, constipation, flatulence, colds, flu, indigestion.

Uses for Women: Frigidity.

Uses for Babies and Children: Use in moderation only.

Use for the Home: Cleaning.

Use for Travel: Minor digestive upsets.

Social and Seasonal Use: Warming, spicy blends.

Ways to Use: Massage oils, diffusers, candles.

Cautions: Use in moderation as it may be irritating in large doses. Black pepper essential oil is often advised against in use with homeopathic treatments.

Cost: $

Peppermint

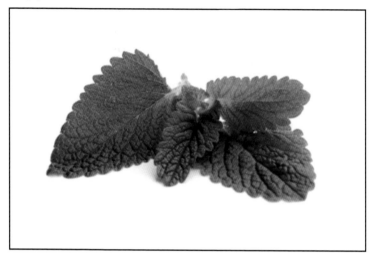

Botanical Name: *Mentha (x) piperita.*

Synonyms: Mint, brandy mint, balm mint.

Botanical Family: *Lamiaceae.*

Note: Top.

Blends Well with: Benzoin, lavender, lemon, mint essential oils, most *Lamiaceae* plant family members.

Alternative Oils: Spearmint (*Mentha spicata*).

Method of Extraction: Steam distillation of the flowering herb.

Distribution of Plant: Peppermint is believed to be a cultivated hybrid of the plant spearmint (*Mentha spicata*) and watermint (*Mentha aquatica*). There are conflicting accounts as to whether the peppermint species used by the ancient Egyptians and Greeks was the same plant that is used today. Modern day peppermint is native to Europe but cultivated in many countries of the world.

Description of Plant: A small, perennial herb that grows up to three feet in height. It has serrated, aromatic, dark-green leaves and tall spikes of purple-colored flowers.

Characteristics of Essential Oil: Pale yellow or pale green in color. It has a strong, minty aroma.

Main Chemical Components of Essential Oil: Alcohols (menthol) and ketones.

Main Therapeutic Properties of Essential Oil: Analgesic, anti-inflammatory, antiseptic, antiviral, astringent, expectorant, emmenagogue, digestive.

Uses for Body Care: Acne, dermatitis.

Uses for Health: Muscle pain, migraines, asthma, bronchitis, colds, flu, mental fatigue, stress, nausea, sinusitis, indigestion.

Uses for Women: Menstrual problems, assists childbirth.

Uses for Babies and Children: Avoid in use with, and around, children and babies.

Use for the Home: Shock, cleaning, first-aid kit.

Use for Travel: Travel sickness, minor digestive problems.

Social and Seasonal Use: Students and work (mental fatigue), conversation starter/social mingling at parties and celebrations.

Ways to Use: Massage oils, diffusers, skin-care bases (scrubs, lotions, creams, butters, balms), sprays, bath products (oils, fizzes, melts, salts), candles. Also available as a hydrosol.

Cautions: Peppermint essential oil contains a high level of menthol and menthone; for this reason, it may cause skin irritation. It is also advisable to keep peppermint essential oil away from young children and babies for the same reason. Avoid in pregnancy as it may stimulate childbirth. Use in moderation.

Cost: $

Petitgrain

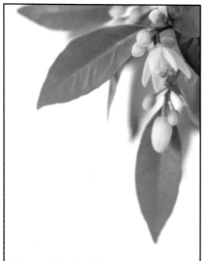

Botanical Name: *Citrus aurantium* var. *amara*.

Synonyms: *Citrus aurantium* var. *bigardia*, petitgrain bigarade, *Citrus aurantium* var. *fol.*

Botanical Family: *Rutaceae*.

Note: Top.

Blends Well with: Lavender, nutmeg, geranium, clary sage, clove, other citrus "orange" oils.

Alternative Oils: Neroli (*Citrus aurantium* var. *amara*), bergamot (*Citrus bergamia*), petitgrain sur fleurs/petitgrain neroli (a distilled blend of both neroil and petitgrain essential oils).

Method of Extraction: Steam distillation of the leaves (and twigs).

Distribution of Plant: Native to China and India; the essential oil is distilled mainly in France and Paraguay.

Description of Plant: An evergreen tree that grows up to thirty-three feet in height. It has glossy, green leaves. The white flowers are aromatic. Petitgrain essential oil is distilled from the bitter orange tree, which also produces neroli essential oil (from the flowers) and bitter orange essential oil (from the fruit).

Characteristics of Essential Oil: Pale yellow in color. It has a fresh, citrus, light floral aroma.

Main Chemical Components of Essential Oil: Esters and alcohols.

Main Therapeutic Properties of Essential Oil: Antiseptic, digestive, antibacterial, anti-inflammatory, balancing, calming.

Uses for Body Care: Oily skin, acne.

Uses for Health: Flatulence, indigestion (stress-related), depression, stress, anxiety, respiratory problems.

Uses for Women: Panic attacks, depression.

Uses for Babies and Children: Skin problems.

Use for the Home: Air fresheners.

Use for Travel: skin-care, stress-related problems.

Social and Seasonal Use: Uplifting blends.

Ways to Use: Massage oils, diffusers, skin-care bases (scrubs, lotions, creams, butters, balms), sprays, bath products (oils, fizzes, melts, salts), candles. Traditional ingredient of eau-de-cologne.

Cautions: No known contraindications for general aromatherapy use.

Cost: $

Pine (Scotch)

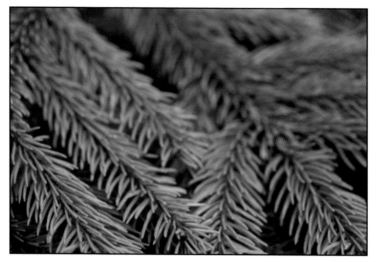

Botanical Name: *Pinus sylvestris.*

Synonyms: Pine, Scots pine, Scots fir, pine needle, Norway pine.

Botanical Family: *Pinaceae.*

Note: Middle.

Blends Well with: Cypress, cedarwood, juniper, lavender, lemon.

Alternative Oils: Silver fir (*Abies alba*), juniper berry (*Juniperus communis*), cypress (*Cupressus sempervirens*).

Method of Extraction: Distillation of the needles.

Distribution of Plant: Native to Europe and Asia. It is now cultivated in Europe, the United States, and Russia.

Description of Plant: A tall, evergreen tree that grows up to 131 feet in height. It has a flat crown. The stiff, long, green needles are paired. It also has brown cones. Pine trees live for hundreds of years.

Characteristics of Essential Oil: Colorless to pale yellow in color. It has a strong, dry, balsamic aroma.

Main Chemical Components of Essential Oil: Monoterpenes.

Main Therapeutic Properties of Essential Oil: Antiseptic, anti-viral, antibacterial, expectorant, decongestant, analgesic.

Uses for Body Care: Eczema, psoriasis.

Uses for Health: Arthritis, muscle pain, asthma, bronchitis, cuts, colds, stress, sinusitis.

Uses for Women: Nervous exhaustion, frigidity.

Uses for Babies and Children: Choose another essential oil in preference.

Use for the Home: Cleaning.

Use for Travel: Respiratory problems.

Social and Seasonal Use: Cleaning yoga mat, cleansing winter blends.

Ways to Use: Massage oils, diffusers, skin-care bases (scrubs, lotions, creams, butters, balms), sprays, candles. Also available as a hydrosol.

Cautions: Avoid if you suffer from skin allergies.

Cost: $

Rose

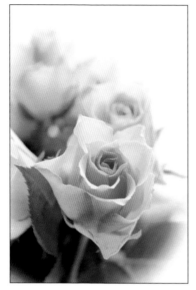

Botanical Name: *Rosa (x) damascena.*

Synonyms: Rose otto, Damask rose, Damascus rose, Turkish rose, Bulgarian rose, rose attar, "queen of flowers."

Botanical Family: *Rosaceae.*

Note: Base.

Blends Well with: Geranium, lavender, frankincense, floral and spice note essential oils.

Alternative Oils: Geranium (*Pelargonium graveolens*), Maroc chamomile (*Ormenis multicaulis*).

Method of Extraction: Steam distillation of the fresh rose petals. An absolute is also produced via solvent extraction.

Distribution of Plant: Roses are native to the Orient, but many species have been cultivated and hybridized. The essential oil is produced in many countries, including France, Bulgaria, and Turkey.

Description of Plant: A small shrub or bush that has sharp thorns and green, pinnate leaves. Rose bushes grow to various heights and sizes, depending upon species. The fragrant flowers of *Rosa (x) damascena* vary from pink to red in color.

Characteristics of Essential Oil: Pale yellow in color with a rich, heady, sweet, floral aroma.

Main Chemical Components of Essential Oil: Alcohols and monoterpenes.

Main Therapeutic Properties of Essential Oil: Antidepressant, aphrodisiac, astringent, sedative, anti-inflammatory, cicatrizant, anti-infectious.

Uses for Body Care: Dry skin, eczema, mature skin, wrinkles, sensitive skin.

Uses for Health: Depression, insomnia, headaches, stress, wounds.

Uses for Women: Irregular menstruation, sexual problems, PMS.

Uses for Babies and Children: Increases confidence, reduces jealousy, excellent for baby skin-care.

Use for the Home: Choose another essential oil in preference.

Use for Travel: General skin-care.

Social and Seasonal Use: Weddings, romantic parties, and celebrations.

Ways to Use: Massage oils, diffusers, skin-care bases (scrubs, lotions, creams, butters, balms), perfume base, sprays, bath products (oils, fizzes, melts, salts), candles. Also available as a hydrosol.

Cautions: No known contraindications for general aromatherapy use. Check to ensure that you are not buying an adulterated version of true rose essential oil.

Cost: $$$

Rosemary

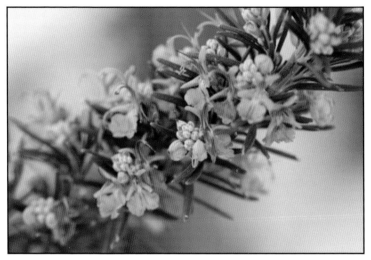

Botanical Name: *Rosmarinus officinalis.*

Synonyms: Incensier (in old French language), *Rosmarinus coronarium*, compass plant.

Botanical Family: *Lamiaceae.*

Note: Middle.

Blends Well with: Lavender, thyme, peppermint, *Lamiaceae* plant family members, spice note essential oils.

Alternative Oils: Common sage (*Salvia officinalis*).

Method of Extraction: Steam distillation of the fresh, flowering tops.

Distribution of Plant: Native to the Mediterranean region. It is now cultivated in many countries, including the United Kingdom and the United States.

Description of Plant: A small herb or shrub that can grow up to six feet in height. It has spiky, needle-shaped leaves that are silver-green in color. It has pale blue, aromatic flowers.

Characteristics of Essential Oil: Pale yellow in color. It has a fresh, camphoraceous aroma with slightly minty undertones. Rosemary essential oil is available as several chemotypes. The main chemotypes are ct. camphor, ct. verbonone, and ct. cineole. Each chemotype will vary slightly in therapeutic properties, depending upon the dominant chemical component.

Main Chemical Components of Essential Oil: Monoterpenes, oxides, and ketones.

Main Therapeutic Properties of Essential Oil: Analgesic, antiseptic, anti-inflammatory, antibacterial, astringent, decongestant, emmenagogue, expectorant.

Uses for Body Care: Acne, dermatitis, eczema.

Uses for Health: Muscle pain, poor circulation, arthritis, rheumatism, asthma, sinusitis, mental fatigue, stimulate memory, coughs and colds.

Uses for Women: Fluid retention, cellulite, amenorrhea.

Uses for Babies and Children: Hair lice (strongly diluted with tea tree essential oil and a shampoo base). Do not use with babies.

Use for the Home: Air fresheners, cleaning.

Use for Travel: Choose another essential oil in preference.

Social and Seasonal Use: In the office to lift mood, increase performance, and stimulate memory; as a study aid for memory; weddings.

Ways to Use: Massage oils, diffusers, skin-care bases (scrubs, lotions, creams, butters, balms), perfume base, sprays, bath products (oils, fizzes, melts, salts), candles. Also available as a hydrosol.

Cautions: Contraindicated for use with high blood pressure. Some sources contraindicate the use of rosemary essential oil in pregnancy and with epilepsy. Use in dilution.

Cost: $

Sandalwood

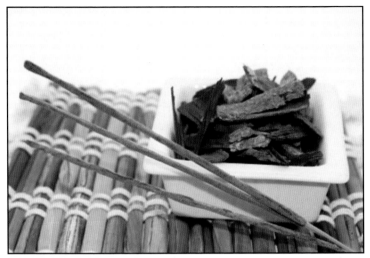

Botanical Name: *Santalum album.*

Synonyms: Sandalwood mysore, East Indian sandalwood (do not confuse with amyris (*Amyris balsamifera*) known as West Indian sandalwood), yellow sandalwood.

Botanical Family: *Santalaceae.*

Note: Base.

Blends Well with: Clove, myrrh, lavender, bergamot, ylang ylang, rose, vetiver.

Alternative Oils: Sandalwood (*Santalum austrocaledonicum*), patchouli (*Pogestemon cablin*).

Method of Extraction: Steam distillation of the heartwood.

Distribution of Plant: Native to tropical Asia. Traditionally, the Mysore region of India produced sandalwood as an essential oil. However, the species *Santalum album* is listed on the IUCN List of Threatened Species (2012.2) as vulnerable. As a consequence, many aromatherapists are seeking an alternative, such as *Santalum austrocaledonicum*, which is chemically similar to *Santalum album* and grown in New Caledonia.

Description of Plant: An evergreen tree that grows up to thirty feet in height. It has small, pink flowers, brown-gray bark, and green, leathery leaves. The essential oil is extracted from the tree when it reaches maturity at thirty years of age.

Characteristics of Essential Oil: Yellow-brown in color with a deep, balsamic-woody aroma. The essential oil is thick in consistency.

Main Chemical Components of Essential Oil: Alcohols.

Main Therapeutic Properties of Essential Oil: Antidepressant, aphrodisiac, antibacterial, decongestant, sedative, anti-infectious, sexual tonic.

Uses for Body Care: Dry, cracked skin, acne, moisturizer.

Uses for Health: Depression, insomnia, stress, sciatica, bronchitis, coughs.

Uses for Women: Varicose veins.

Uses for Babies and Children: Skin care.

Use for the Home: Bereavement.

Use for Travel: Sunburn.

Social and Seasonal Use: Yoga practice, meditation, weddings, romantic parties and celebrations.

Ways to Use: Massage oils, diffusers, skin-care bases (scrubs, lotions, creams, butters, balms), perfume base, sprays, bath products (oils, fizzes, melts, salts), candles. Also available as a hydrosol.

Cautions: No known contraindications in general aromatherapy use. Alternative species of sandalwood essential oil, in addition to those mentioned above, include Royal Hawaiian (*Santalum paniculatum*) and Australian (*Santalum spicta*). Check for the latest information on these alternatives before using them to see if they are currently viable.

Cost: $$$

Tea Tree

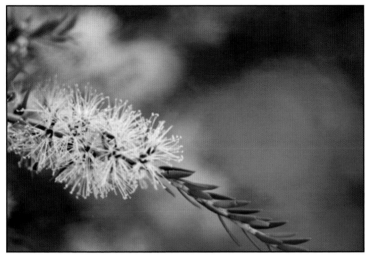

Botanical Name: *Melaleuca alternifolia*

Synonyms: Ti-tree, narrow-leaved (paperbark) tea tree.

Botanical Family: *Myrtaceae.*

Note: Top.

Blends Well with: Lemon, lavender, clove, geranium.

Alternative Oils: Sweet marjoram (*Origanum marjorana*), Spanish sage (*Salvia lavandulifolia*).

Method of Extraction: Steam distillation of the leaves and twigs.

Distribution of Plant: Native to Australia. There are other varieties of plants called tea tree, but only the species *Melaleuca alternifolia* produces true tea tree essential oil.

Description of Plant: A small tree with needle-like, gray-green leaves and small flowers on spikes.

Characteristics of Essential Oil: Pale yellow in color, with a strong, antiseptic, camphoraceous aroma.

Main Chemical Components of Essential Oil: Alcohols and monoterpenes.

Main Therapeutic Properties of Essential Oil: Antiseptic, anti-infectious, antiviral, anti-inflammatory, antibacterial, immuno-stimulant, analgesic.

Uses for Body Care: Oily skin, acne, rashes.

Uses for Health: Burns, infections, infected wounds, asthma, bronchitis, colds, fever, cold sores (herpes).

Uses for Women: Candida.

Uses for Babies and Children: Chicken pox, hair lice (strongly diluted with rosemary or lavender essential oil and a shampoo base).

Use for the Home: Cleaning, laundry, first-aid kit.

Use for Travel: Insect bites.

Social and Seasonal Use: Cleaning yoga mat, cleansing blends.

Ways to Use: Massage oils, diffusers, skin-care bases (scrubs, lotions, creams, butters, balms), sprays, candles. Also available as a hydrosol.

Cautions: Possible sensitization on the skin, even in dilution; take care with babies and children.

Cost: $

Thyme

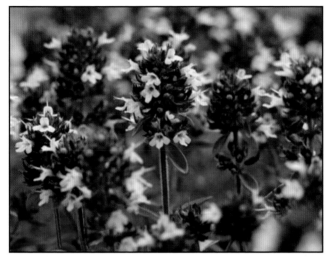

Botanical Name: *Thymus vulgaris.*

Synonyms: (Depending upon distillate and chemotype) French thyme, white thyme, common thyme, red thyme.

Botanical Family: *Lamiaceae.*

Note: Top.

Blends Well with: Rosemary, lemon, bergamot, lavender, geranium.

Alternative Oils: Moroccan thyme (*Thymus satureioides*), basil (*Ocimum basilicum*).

Method of Extraction: Distillation of the flowering tops and leaves.

Distribution of Plant: Native to the Mediterranean region. It is now cultivated in several places, including the United States and central Europe.

Description of Plant: A perennial, evergreen herb that grows up to two feet in height. It has small, oval, green leaves and purple or white flowers.

Characteristics of Essential Oil: Red thyme—red-brown in color with a slightly spicy, herbaceous aroma. It has green undertones. White thyme—pale yellow in color with a sweet, green aroma.

Main Chemical Components of Essential Oil: Phenols, alcohols, and monoterpenes (depending upon chemotype; see note below).

Main Therapeutic Properties of Essential Oil: Antiseptic, astringent, antibacterial, antimicrobial.

Uses for Body Care: Eczema, acne, dermatitis, bruises.

Uses for Health: Burns, arthritis, muscle pain, asthma, bronchitis, colds, flatulence, headaches.

Uses for Women: Avoid in pregnancy.

Uses for Babies and Children: Choose another essential oil in preference.

Use for the Home: Air fresheners, cleaning.

Use for Travel: Choose another essential oil in preference.

Social and Seasonal Use: Cleaning yoga mat, cleansing blends.

Ways to Use: Massage oils, diffusers, skin-care bases (scrubs, lotions, creams, butters, balms), sprays, candles. Also available as a hydrosol.

Cautions: Avoid in use with high blood pressure or pregnancy.

Cost: $

Special Note:

Red thyme is distilled from the crude distillate of this plant, whereas white thyme is the refined distillation (second distillate) of red thyme. Thyme produces several chemotypes, including *Thymus vulgaris* ct. thymol, *Thymus vulgaris* ct. carvacrol, *Thymus vulgaris* ct. linalool, and *Thymus vulgaris* ct. thujanal—4. Sometimes, the former two varieties are referred to as red thyme, and the latter two varieties referred to as white thyme—although this can be confusing. *Thymus vulgaris* ct. thymol and *Thymus vulgaris* ct.

carvacrol contain a higher level of phenols; *Thymus vulgaris* ct. linalool and *Thymus vulgaris* ct. thujanal—4 contain a higher level of alcohols. In general, the former chemotypes specified will be more aggressive in nature than the latter chemotypes specified. These varying chemical components will reflect a differentiation in the therapeutic properties of each oil, too. Therefore, this reference guide should be referred to in general terms, depending upon both the thyme distillate and chemotype used.

Vetiver

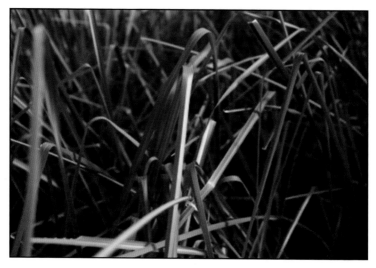

Botanical Name: *Vetiveria zizanioides.*

Synonyms: Vetivert, khus khus, *Andropogon muricatus.*

Botanical Family: *Poaceae.*

Note: Base.

Blends Well with: Sandalwood, sweet orange, lavender, geranium, patchouli, jasmine.

Alternative Oils: Peppermint (*Mentha piperita*), cedarwood (*Cedrus atlantica*).

Method of Extraction: Steam distillation from the roots. The distillation process is labor intensive, as the roots have to be dug and washed before being slowly distilled.

Distribution of Plant: Native to Indonesia, Sri Lanka, and southern India. It is now cultivated in countries with a similar climate and growing conditions.

Description of Plant: A perennial, scented grass with long, narrow leaves. It has a complicated root system. Vetiver is botanically related to citronella.

Characteristics of Essential Oil: Olive or amber in color. It has a smoky, earthy aroma that is slightly woody, too.

Main Chemical Components of Essential Oil: Alcohols and ketones.

Main Therapeutic Properties of Essential Oil: Antiseptic, sedative, calming, stimulant to the circulatory and immune systems, aphrodisiac.

Uses for Body Care: Oily skin, acne.

Uses for Health: Wounds, arthritis, rheumatism, muscle pain, insomnia, depression, stress.

Uses for Women: Amenorrhea.

Uses for Babies and Children: Use with caution due to ketones content.

Use for the Home: Shock, bereavement.

Use for Travel: To calm in stressful situations.

Social and Seasonal Use: Yoga practice, relaxation blends at parties and celebrations.

Ways to Use: Massage oils, diffusers, skin-care bases (scrubs, lotions, creams, butters, balms), perfume base, sprays, bath products (oils, fizzes, melts, salts), candles. Also available as a hydrosol.

Cautions: No known contraindications for general aromatherapy use.

Cost: $$

Yarrow

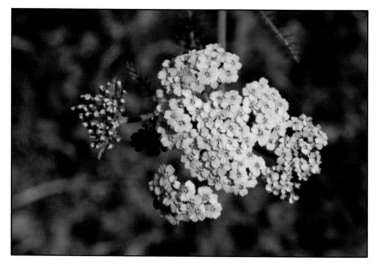

Botanical Name: *Achillea millefolium.*

Synonyms: Milfoil, old man's pepper, thousand leaf, nose bleed, devil's nettle, bloodwort, yarroway.

Botanical Family: *Asteraceae.*

Note: Middle.

Blends Well with: Clove, cedarwood, chamomile, vetiver.

Alternative Oils: Black pepper (*Piper nigrum*), myrrh (*Commiphora myrrha*), patchouli (*Pogostemon cablin*).

Method of Extraction: Steam distillation of the flowerheads.

Distribution of Plant: Native to Europe and Asia. It is now cultivated in countries with a similar climate and growing conditions, including the United States.

Description of Plant: A perennial herb that grows up to three feet in height. It has feathery-looking leaves with pink-white or mauve flowers.

Characteristics of Essential Oil: Dark blue or green in color. It has a sweet, green, herbaceous-camphoraceous aroma.

Main Chemical Components of Essential Oil: Sesquiterpenes and monoterpenes.

Main Therapeutic Properties of Essential Oil: Anti-inflammatory, antiseptic, astringent, digestive, expectorant, emmenagogue.

Uses for Body Care: Eczema, acne, scars, skin toning.

Uses for Health: Wounds, rheumatoid arthritis, colds, insomnia, indigestion, constipation, hemorrhoids, stress.

Uses for Women: Dysmenorrhea, amenorrhea.

Uses for Babies and Children: Choose another essential oil in preference.

Use for the Home: First-aid kit.

Use for Travel: Minor digestive problems.

Social and Seasonal Use: Cleansing blends.

Ways to Use: Massage oils, diffusers, skin-care bases (scrubs, lotions, creams, butters, balms), sprays, candles. Also available as a hydrosol.

Cautions: Use in moderation as it may cause skin sensitization. Avoid in use with young children and in pregnancy.

Cost: $$$

Ylang Ylang

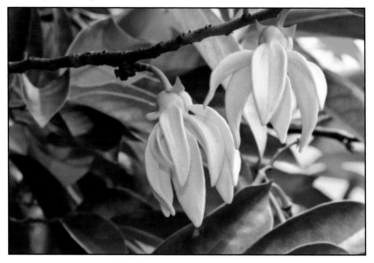

Botanical Name: *Cananga odorata.*

Synonyms: Flower of flowers, *Unona odaratissimum* (there are several variations on this particular synonym).

Botanical Family: *Annonaceae.*

Note: Base.

Blends Well with: Sweet orange, lavender, geranium, lemon, bergamot, sandalwood, jasmine.

Alternative Oils: Patchouli (*Pogestomon cablin*), myrrh (*Commiphora myrrha*).

Method of Extraction: Steam distillation of the fresh flowers. Distillation is slow and complex and is sometimes sold as separate (part of) distillates. The complete distillate is the recommended distillate for aromatherapy use.

Distribution of Plant: Native to tropical Asia, including the Philippines and Indonesia. It is now cultivated in various other countries for essential oil production.

Description of Plant: A tropical tree or bush with large flowers that are white, yellow, or pink in color. It grows up to a height of sixty-five feet.

Characteristics of Essential Oil: Pale yellow in color, with a sweet, intoxicating, floral aroma.

Main Chemical Components of Essential Oil: Sesquiterpenes, alcohols, esters, and phenols.

Main Therapeutic Properties of Essential Oil: Antiseptic, aphrodisiac, antidepressant, balancing, calming, sedative, and stimulant to the reproductive system.

Uses for Body Care: Oily skin, acne, general skin-care.

Uses for Health: Depression, insomnia, stress.

Uses for Women: Frigidity, hair rinse.

Uses for Babies and Children: Skin care, anxiety, hyperactivity, temper tantrums.

Use for the Home: Shock.

Use for Travel: Anxiety related to travel.

Social and Seasonal Use: Weddings, romantic blends for parties and celebrations.

Ways to Use: Massage oils, diffusers, skin-care bases (scrubs, lotions, creams, butters, balms), perfume base, sprays, bath products (oils, fizzes, melts, salts), candles.

Cautions: May cause headaches or nausea if used in large quantities.

Cost: $

Bibliography

"3-1-1 for Carry-ons," www.tsa.gov/traveler-information/3-1-1-carry-ons

"About IUCN," www.iucn.org/about/.

"Argan Oil: A Great Source of Natural Gamma-Tocopherol, Unsaturated Fatty Acids, Squalene and Sterols." Antanais Corp (Suisse) SA, www.fda.gov/ohrms/dockets/dockets/95s0316/95s-0316-rpt0255-05-Argan-Oil-vol174.pdf.

"Aromatherapy," www.med.nyu.edu/content?ChunkIID=37427.

"Attar of Roses," www.britannica.com/EBchecked/topic/42117/attar-of-roses.

Bell, Kristen Leigh, *Holistic Aromatherapy for Animals* (Scotland: Findhorn Press, 2002).

Brown, Denise Whichello, *Teach Yourself Massage* (London: Bookpoint Ltd, 2003).

Buckle, Jane, *Clinical Aromatherapy: Essential Oils in Practice*, 2nd ed. (London: Churchill Livingstone, 2003).

Burfield, Tony, "Updated List of Threatened Aromatic Plants Used in the Aroma and Cosmetic Industries," Cropwatch 1, no. 21 (March 2010), www.cropwatch.org/Threatened%20Aromatic%20Species%20v1.21.pdf.

Clarke, Sue, *Essential Chemistry for Aromatherapy* (London: Churchill Livingstone, 2008).

"Distillation Kits," www.copperstills.com/index.php/9-uncategorised/35-kits.

Duckett, P., et al., "Aromas of Rosemary and Lavender Essential Oils Differentially Affect Cognition and Mood in Healthy Adults." *International Journal of Neuroscience* 13, no. 1

(2003): 15–38, www.ncbi.nlm.nih.gov/pubmed/?term=ros
emary+essential+oil+for+memory.

"Extraction Methods of Natural Essential Oils," Tamil Nadu
Agricultural University, India,http://agritech.tnau.ac.in/
horticulture/extraction_methods_natural_essential_oil.pdf.

de Feydeau, Elisabeth, *A Scented Palace* (London: I. B. Tauris & Co.
Ltd, 2006).

de Feydeau, Elisabeth, *Les Parfums: Histoire, Anthologie, Dictionnaire*
(Paris: Bouquins, 2011).

Fleischer, "Untersuchungen uber das Reabsorptionsvermögen
der Menschlichen Haut," *ErlangenHabilitatsionsschrift*,
(1877): 81.

Giordano, Carlo, and Angelandrea Casale, *Profumi, Unguenti e
Acconciature in Pompei Antica* (Rome: Bardi Editore, 1992).

Grieve, M., "Roses: A Modern Herbal," www.botanical.com/
botanical/mgmh/r/roses-18.html.

"How Lavender Oil Is Made," www.auracacia.com/auracacia/
aclearn/features/lavender3.html.

International Journal of Clinical Aromatherapy Paediatrics Care 2, no.
2 (2005).

Jäger, W., et al., "Percutaneous Absorption of Lavender Oil from
a Massage Oil," *J. Soc. Cosmet. Chem.* 43, no. 1 (1992): 49–54.

Keville, Kathi, and Mindy Green, *Aromatherapy: A Complete Guide
to the Healing Art*, 2nd ed. (New York: Crown Publishing,
2009).

Kiecolt-Glaser J.K., et al., "Olfactory Influences on Mood
and Autonomic, Endocrine, and Immune Function,"
Psychoneuroendocrinology 33, no. 3 (2008): 328–39,
www. ncbi.nlm.nih.gov/pubmed/18178322.

Lawless, Julia, *The Illustrated Encyclopedia of Essential Oils* (London: Element, 1995).

———. *The Aromatherapy Garden* (London: Kyle Cathie Ltd., 2001).

Moss, M. et al., "Modulation of Cognitive Performance and Mood by Aromas of Peppermint and Ylang Ylang," *Int. J. Neurosci.* 118, no. 1 (2008): 59–77, www.ncbi.nlm.nih.gov/pubmed/18041606.

Moss M., J. Cook, K. Wesnes, and P. Duckett, "Aromas of Rosemary and Lavender Essential Oils Differentially Affect Cognition and Mood in Healthy Adults," Int. J. Neurosci. 113, no. 1 (2003): 15–38, http://www.ncbi.nlm.nih.gov/pubmed/12690999.

National Association for Holistic Aromatherapy, PO Box 27871, Raleigh, NC, 27611-7871, United States.

"Organic Farming and Labeling," www.usda.gov/wps/portal/usda/usdahome?navid=ORGANIC_CERTIFICATIO.

Oxford English Dictionary, 10th ed. (UK: Oxford University Press, 1999).

Penny Price Academy of Aromatherapy, Spa Villa, 41 Leicester Road, Hinckley, LE10 1LW, Leicestershire, England.

Rose, J. E., and F. M. Behm, "Inhalation of Vapor from Black Pepper Extract Reduces Smoking Withdrawal Symptoms," *Drug Alcohol Depend* 34, no. 3 (1994): 225–9, www.ncbi.nlm.nih.gov/pubmed/8033760.

van der Ploeg, Eva S. et al., "The Study Protocol of a Blinded Randomised-Controlled Cross-Over Trial of Lavender Oil as a Treatment of Behavioral Symptoms in Dementia," (2010), www.biomedcentral.com/1471-2318/10/49.

Price, Shirley, *Aromatherapy Workbook*, (UK: Thorsons, 2000).

———. *Aromatherapy for Women* (UK: Southwater, 2003).

Price, Shirley, and Len Price, *Aromatherapy for Health Professionals* 4th ed. (UK: Churchill Livingstone, 2012).

Price, Shirley, and Penny Price, *Aromatherapy for Babies and Children*, (UK: Riverhead, 1996).

"Research, Education, and Promotion of Hydrosols," www.circle-hinstitute.com/index.php/hydrosol-information.

Scheffer, Mechthild, *The Encyclopedia of Bach Flower Therapy*, (US: Healing Arts Press, 2001).

Tildesley, N. T., et al., "Positive Modulation of Mood and Cognitive Performance Following Administrative Doses of Salvia lavandulaefolia Essential Oil," *Physiol. Behav.* 17, no. 5 (2005): 699–709, www.ncbi.nlm.nih.gov/pubmed/15639154.

Valette, G., and E. Sobrin, "Percutaneous Absorption of Various Animal and Vegetable Oils," *Pharmica Acta Helvetica* 38, no. 10 (1963), 710–716.

Waugh, Ann, and Allison Grant, *Ross and Wilson Anatomy and Physiology in Health and Illness*, 9th ed. (UK: Churchill Livingstone, 2001).

Worwood, Valerie Ann, *The Complete Book of Essential Oils and Aromatherapy*, (California: New World Library, 1991).

Recommended Resources

The following companies and distributors are a few of my recommended resources for essential oils, carrier oils, and other ingredients for aromatherapy use, based on personal experience and/or knowledge of the supplier. Although several of these companies carry a wide range of supplies, I have categorized them on personal use (and recommendation) of those particular products mentioned.

Be aware that information is subject to change, so check for up-to-date information before contacting them.

Essential Oils and Carrier Oils:

Penny Price Aromatherapy
Spa Villa
41 Leicester Road
Hinckley
LE10 1LW
UK

Phone: (0844) 8844-966
Website: www.penny-price.com
Recommended for: Essential oils, carrier oils, hydrosols, and all supplies

Penny Price essential oils are available to customers in the United States by contacting Sharon Falsetto at Sedona Aromatherapie:

Website: www.sedonaaromatherapie.com
Email: sharon@sedonaaromatherapie.com

The Jojoba Company
P.O. Box 586
Waldoboro, ME
04572

Phone: (1-800) 256-5622
Website: www.jojobacompany.com
Email: hobacare@jojobacompany.com
Recommended for: Jojoba oil

Home Distillation Kits:

IAG Botanics LLC
USA

Phone: (509) 722-3150
Website: www. copperstills.com
Recommended for: High
quality copper stills

Other Aromatherapy Ingredients and Supplies:

From Nature with Love
Natural Sourcing LLC
341 Christian Street
Oxford, CT 06478

Phone: (1-800) 520-2060
Website: www.fromnature-
withlove.com
Recommended for: Butters,
salts, and sugars

Aromatics International
9280 Mormon Creek Road
Lolo, MT
59847

Phone: (406) 273-9833
Website: www.aromaticsinter-
national.com
Recommended for: Especially
beeswax

Candle Science
2700 Perimeter Park Drive
Suite 150
Morrisville, NC
27560

Phone: (1-888) 266-3916
Website: www.candlescience.com
Email: support@candle-
science.com
Recommended for: Soy candle
wax

Index